FABhealth

Praise for FAB Health

"Paulette Agnew's book *FAB Health* is a practical and yet intriguing look into the power of energy to heal the body, whether that energy comes from the sun, water, food, bio-energetic devices or any other healing modality. We are all composed of energy, and every outside source of energy, whether from harmful manmade electromagnetic fields, or healing therapies, affects the energy of every single cell in our bodies, for better or for worse.

Paulette provides amazing insights into how natural, common things that we take for granted—things like the sun, ions from a rainstorm or waterfall, the earth beneath our feet, and healthy food—can do wonders for rejuvenating the body. She explains on an energetic and biochemical level, *how* and *why* these things affect the body's innate energy field. In so doing, she provides motivation and inspiration for those of us who have become numb to the detrimental effects of Wi-Fi and an artificial, polluted lifestyle indoors, to go back to the basics and find better and yet simpler ways to be well with the tools God has given us.

What's more, as someone who had a severe case of chronic Lyme disease and yet recovered using bioenergetic medicine, Paulette provides hope to the even the sickest of the sick with Lyme. Her story is a testimony to the fact that bioenergetic medicine is effective for healing even the most insidious degenerative diseases— without negative side effects. This should give hope to those who have failed antibiotic or other conventional therapies. Antibiotics, while useful, don't always work for everyone and often leave more damage in their wake so better alternatives like those found in energy medicine are much needed. I highly recommend Paulette's book to people with Lyme and those with chronic degenerative disease, as well as to those who simply want to better their health with tools that truly work."

Connie Strasheim,
Author, *New Paradigms in Lyme Disease Treatment: 10 Top Doctors Reveal Healing Strategies that Work* and 10 other books on holistic wellness

---

"As people get sicker and sicker from toxins, superbugs, Lyme's Disease, cancer, etc. astonishing opportunities arise. On one side: opportunities to question the very paradigms that got us sick in the first place. And on the other side: opportunities for new strategies for healing. Those of us who have battled for our own health and the health of our loved ones—and won—know that our civilization's health systems are really disease systems and lack the insight, inspiration and innovation necessary to aid those most in need. Materialistic chemistry is sold to us by medical schools, doctors and gigantic corporations as the forefront of science yet materialistic chemistry's prize: the pill, hasn't solved our ills. As Paulette Agnew details in her book, FAB Health, a new type of medicine is already here and it has been gaining momentum. This new medicine, or as Agnew calls it, FAB Medicine (Frequency and Bioenergetic Medicine) includes light, energy, frequency and electromagnetic treatments for reversing poor health and infections. FAB Medicine can be utilized with other treatments providing a better, more diverse strategy for healing. Paulette Agnew's book FAB Health arrives just in time and for you, the reader, can be a life saver."

David 'Avocado' Wolfe,

nutritionist, adventurer, organic / biodynamic farmer, www.davidwolfe.com, www.facebook.com/ DavidAvocadoWolfe, author of The Beauty Diet, founder of the non-profit www.ftpf.org.

"I really enjoyed this book; it's so interesting and dense, it presents a wide array of modalities of healing and at the same time replete with common sense. Paulette has managed to paint a picture for the reader a glimpse of the future of medicine or where medicine needs to be heading. In so few pages, she has introduced us to the physics and the chemistry of healing with herself as the living evidence of its efficacy. I found myself agreeing wholeheartedly to so many of the things Paulette wrote, none less than the fact that to improve health one needs to change one's lifestyle, one's diet and one's attitude! Paulette Agnew provides a roadmap towards better health, especially for anyone with a chronic condition such as Lyme Disease. With regret, there's a big audience that needs this book but happily this book is here for that large audience."

Antony Haynes,

Registered Nutritional Therapist, Functional Medicine Practitioner, Author, Lecturer, Teacher, Mentor

---

"If you are struggling with Lyme disease or Chronic Fatigue Syndrome, you definitely need to check out this book. I appreciate the holistic approach this book recommends for those struggling with challenging health conditions. Paulette takes you on her personal journey of healing and is living proof that this approach works."

Dr. Laura Ricci,

PT, DPT, NBC-HWC, WHNC

"Paulette Agnew's book provides us with a much-needed explanation of why we get sick—at a molecular level—but also how we can regain health, especially when dealing with serious illness. This is a priceless wealth of information and a gateway to a new era of health self-management.

This labour of love is packed with invaluable research and cutting-edge concepts that will bring new understanding—and hope—to anyone dealing with serious illness. Essential reading if you care about your health. It really is a manual for living constructively at a cellular level—I couldn't put it down."

Margaret Cahill,
Author, *Under Cover of Darkness: How I Blogged My Way Through Mantle Cell Lymphoma.*

"What a GENIUS explanation of our bioelectric body and the new paradigm of medicine that is emerging! I love how Paulette shares from her personal experience as well as from the scientific literature to help the reader have a true understanding of how we heal and what can be done to assist this. For doctors, practitioners, and individuals, this book is a packed with insight and information about this new medical paradigm and how to apply it now."

Kim D'Eramo,
D.O., Founder of The American Institute of Mind Body Medicine

---

"*FAB Health* is an important book in the field of holistic healing and naturopathic medicine and should be on the bookshelf of every holistic practitioner."

Antony J. Edwards,
ND MD (MA) Psychotherapy MANM FBIH FRCP (MA)

"*FAB Health* is both well written and profound as it challenges so much of what we know about medical research. Paulette Agnew skilfully leads us into understanding a whole new healing possibility, which could become an important part of mainstream medicine in the next ten years. All patients, their lives, surroundings and history are different and require an integrated approach to healing. This book goes a long way towards enlightening us all about the real cause of illness, and shows us the way back to complete health through simple and natural solutions, especially with the rise of superbugs. If everyone read this book and embraced even a few of Paulette's concepts, there would be a much less strain on our health care systems."

M. Erik,
MD, PhD, Netherlands

"FAB is clearly an important healing modality that has enormous potential for the future. Conventional medicine is in an unacknowledged crisis of sustainability and FAB offers an approach that is genuinely capable of creating health rather than simply fighting disease."

Robert A Duddell,
BA MARH Homeopath.

"I love this book! It gives a beautiful explanation of how energy works and healing occurs. Paulette uses herself as the model of how FAB works and is effective. Her explanations are understandable and lay the foundation for the future of medicine in a clear concise way. Please read it!"

Shiroko Sokitch,
MD, Heart to Heart Medical Center

"An eye-opening book which combines the natural, such as walking barefoot and catching the sun's rays now and again, with the latest high-tech advances in creating wellness and fighting disease. The scientific explanations are thoroughly well researched and backed up by the author's personal experiences. The future is here—a must-read for all medical practitioners and everyone who wants to keep well."

Piers Warren,
Author and Principal of *Wildeye: The International School of Wildlife Film-making*

"*FAB Health* is a fabulous journey into Nature's perspectives of human health overlooked by today's current medical model. Founded on science and the vital importance of the body electric, Paulette Agnew shares fascinating and crystal-clear insights on bioenergy and its relationships with health and disease. Here, you can't help but find gems of wisdom that can shape your life and future health."

Jack Tips,
Wellness Wiz

"This is an important book that holds many of the answers to curing Lyme Disease. It certainly had me questioning much of the traditional science and medicine that we were taught at Dental School."

Kevin Lawlor,
Mountain Leader and Wilderness Medic

"*FAB Health* holds our hands in sharing the truth about Health and Dis-ease. Paulette has done a remarkable job in researching, presenting and sharing the knowledge about Bioenergetic and Frequency tools available in Europe. Embracing them requires a paradigm shift but an exciting one that accelerates our journey to wellness. Through her book, we can finally understand the science and reason behind healing. Energy is everything and when we receive its help, now from the assistance of this book and associated lifestyle changes, we come back into energetic flow and balance. I hope someday this book is in every home, for it is about Us and the joy, passions and happiness that health creates in our life."

Dean Martens,
Clinical Herbalist, Founder and President of Herbs of Light Inc.

"*FAB Health* brings you a fabulous life again. When you really do apply the profound selected information to your life, a lot will change. Not only your health will change, but you will experience the full potential of your existence. Paulette managed to bring all the different elements of many different healing techniques together which are well researched and self-explored. It's a real breakthrough for the worldwide bacteria problem."

Raymond Niemeijer,
Clinical Psycho-Neuro-Immunologist, Natural Health Therapist, Physiotherapist, Life-Coach, Yoga teacher and founder of Life-Centre Holland.

"Wildly inspiring! An essential life manual for those of you wishing to radiate health & vitality from the very core of your soul."

Tamara Bell,
ND, Dip., Hom., Naturopath, Homeopath

"*FAB Health*—a very impressive explanation of Frequency and Bioenergy. Not just well researched but valuable information for all. An inspiring must read book for everyone who wants to stay healthy."

Bindi Desai,
Bio-Protective Systems-Living with EMF Radiation

"Paulette Agnew is a powerful and gifted writer who has created a brilliantly organized and essential book for anyone interested in maintaining robust health through understanding the body electric. This book has enabled me to see and understand how my body works on finer and finer levels. By the way, the chapter on Magnetism is a must read! I have already incorporated many of her modalities into my daily routine and I can testify that they make a tremendous positive difference not only for me, but also for my entire family!"

Tina Erwin,
Commander US Navy (Ret) Author and Podcast Host on The Karmic Path

---

"At our clinic, we utilise nearly every bioenergy hack that Paulette mentions in this book. We use them because they work and Paulette's efforts to educate people to see practitioners who use these technologies is right on. With the methods that she describes, we are able to help cure the sick person to reorient the energies in their body toward healthy vibrational relationships. If you are sick, take this book and its information to heart. There is truth here. It is a truth that if acted upon, can not only set you free from disease, but also free to live a happy energetic full life."

David I Minkoff MD,
Lifeworks Wellness Center, Clearwater, FL

"Paulette's clear and humorous explanation of healing process challenges us to think outside the box. Her enthusiasm and passion encouraged me to become more fearless in exploring these possibilities for my patients and myself. Paulette shows how energy and frequency medicine has already been well researched for the last few decades. Yes, caution and research has undoubtedly its place. However, healing the body is not done by pills alone. And as Paulette states, the era of antibiotics might come to grinding halt. Therefore I'm very grateful for all her work and zest she puts into trying to get everybody work together, (complementary and allopathic medicine) for the good of mankind and the world.

"Her book is an eye opener for a more holistic and individual way of treating patients. My dream is to see mainstream hospitals adding this exciting FAB medicine paradigm to give each patient the best chance of restoring health. I agree with Paulette that this could well be the best way forward in the future. Paulette is a true pioneer and deserves our curious and fearless attention to explore new paths of healing."

Dr. Irene ten Berge
MD, Netherlands, GP for 24 years

"I love this book, it is very well written and structured, going through the journey of Paulette's illnesses and her full recovery, explaining the different ways to the well-being and the healing path. It is also a data driven and scientific guide that I would recommend to everyone to read in order understand the basics of FAB leading to a healthy and happy life. Thanks Paulette for putting this piece of art together!"

Migdo Pomar Natal,
Industrial Engineer, Homeopath, Reiki Master & Shamanic Healer

---

"In *FAB Health*, Paulette combines cutting edge research into frequency, vibration and magnetism with the study of the intricate workings and minutiae of cells and organs to arrive at a natural and holistic view. There is something innately satisfying in the use of modern technology with the age-old efficacy of natural healing. This book is a marvellous synthesis of these precepts and is brim full of information for the maintenance of good health. It is down to earth, common sense and easy to read. For those who find themselves in a hopeless state as a result of chronic illness and disease this book is an inspiration. It represents a resounding "Hallelujah!", an oasis in the desert, a practical panacea which is at once healing and self-empowering. I heartily recommend this book."

DarPan

HEALING LYME DISEASE AND OTHER
ILLNESSES WITHOUT ANTIBIOTICS

FAB
health

*Understanding Why We Become Ill
So We Can Get Better*

PAULETTE AGNEW

NEW YORK

LONDON • NASHVILLE • MELBOURNE • VANCOUVER

FABhealth

Understanding Why We Become Ill So We Can Get Better

HEALING LYME DISEASE AND OTHER ILLNESSES WITHOUT ANTIBIOTICS

Published in New York, New York, by Morgan James Publishing. Morgan James is a trademark of Morgan James, LLC. www.MorganJamesPublishing.com

The Morgan James Speakers Group can bring authors to your live event. For more information or to book an event visit The Morgan James Speakers Group at www.TheMorganJamesSpeakersGroup.com.

ISBN 9781683508618 paperback
ISBN 9781683508625 eBook
Library of Congress Control Number: 2017918186

Illustrations by:
Chris Ion
www.chrisionart.co.uk

Cover Design by:
Rachel Lopez
www.r2cdesign.com

Interior Design by:
Christopher Kirk
www.GFSstudio.com

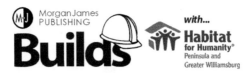

In an effort to support local communities, raise awareness and funds, Morgan James Publishing donates a percentage of all book sales for the life of each book to Habitat for Humanity Peninsula and Greater Williamsburg.

Get involved today! Visit
www.MorganJamesBuilds.com

Also by Paulette Agnew

Beyond Fatigue Online Programme

Traya's Quest (A Spiritual Odyssey for Children)

For more information and other books in the FAB series visit:
www.pauletteagnew.com

Dedication

This book is dedicated to: All the mothers, grandmothers, women and girls and especially my mother Cynthia, an extraordinary, life-long, best friend, mentor and role model. Thank you to the Great Mother Earth for hosting us all and to the Mother of Creation which resides in all, for all time. Your strength, wisdom and love sustains humanity.

Table of Contents

Foreword
By Sir Julian Rose

The rapid acceleration of startling break-throughs in the world of natural medicine and alternative treatments would seem to bear testimony to the fact that we are entering into a period of 'health enlightenment'. Millions worldwide are dumping Big Pharma and seeking a natural cure for ailments that, not long ago, were considered only curable via the operation theatre and months of intensive antibiotic prescriptions.

No longer. In her bubbling and illuminating investigations, Paulette Agnew flings open the window onto a whole new world of non-toxic treatments that aim to bring into harmony cutting edge technological advances and the time-honoured, grandmotherly wisdom of the ages. The light literally pours in—as one shares with Paulette her metamorphosis from someone on the edge of death to a state of full recovery into the joyous fullness of a life to be lived.

A highly persuasive argument that rings out throughout this book points us towards recognition of the holistic nature of our universe, ourselves and all life on our planet. The author leaps boldly into quantum mechanics, demonstrating how every factor of universal energy plays its role in the health and welfare of the billions of intelligent cells that comprise our living organism: body, mind and spirit. It's challenging stuff—and I applaud the placing of such wisdom at the core of the text. Paulette states:

"This concept, our interconnection with all things, could be one of the greatest mysteries of life waiting for each of us to explore. The discovery of our entanglement and the responsibility that lies inherent within this knowledge must be the next step for humanity if we are to survive as a species."

Here is the essential truth that has alluded mankind for so long. A truth which has been blocked by a system that is based on division, separation and tunnel vision decision making. That is where we are today. In politics, economics, education and yes, health care. But, as Bob Dylan noted back in 1962 "The Times They Are A Changin" and, even as the stagnant status quo flounders and fragments around us, we humans are grasping the nettle of something altogether greater and more purposeful.

We are becoming conscious; as Paulette says in the book "The vast majority of people live disconnected from this truth. They may think one thing and say something else, and their hearts have yet another desire and need. Healing is also bringing us back to this state of coherence."

The healing process is indeed about coherence. Quantum coherence. It is about getting into balance all the unbalanced elements of our bodies and our minds. In FAB Health, we learn how the dance of photons and electrons can illuminate the pathways to health; how recharged negative ions spring to the defence of our immune systems; how new technical innovations can channel vibrational energies to revivify failing organs—and how sustained positive thinking and a local, fresh, 'real food' living diet, top all outside interventions.

I warmly recommend entering boldly into the adventure which lies ahead of you amongst the pages of this empowering book. You will come out the other end refreshed—positively hopping with bioenergetic inspiration—and increasingly eager to take-on new levels of self-empowerment.

Sir Julian Rose

Pioneer of organic farming, UK, international activist, author of *In Defense of Life*, advocate for holistic practices

Introduction

This book was inspired by a personal journey from being afflicted by a so-called incurable illness to a full recovery. It is based on my own experiences, as well as my research done over a period of three years.

In the latter stage of my illness, I came across a Frequency and Bioenergy (FAB) practitioner who applies a unique system of Frequency (via devices) alongside herbs, supplements, acupuncture and other natural therapies to treat patients. I soon realised that the combination of FAB treatments combined with changes to one's lifestyle can beat the toughest of infections. After two years of clinical and home-based treatments, without the use of antibiotics or other pharmaceutical drugs, I completely recovered from chronic Lyme Borreliosis.

I was determined to find out how it all works and am now sharing my findings with you in this book.

This book is packed with layers of information, ideas and cutting-edge concepts. It aims to show you that complex health challenges can be understood with a clear and simple approach. You will first learn about the existence of your holographic body, the invisible world of electrons, photons, frequency and energy flow. Through this knowledge, we then explore how illness can arise when a disturbance happens at these levels. Frequency and Bioenergy (FAB) treatments and technology can enhance and balance this layer of life, aiding the healing process.

Although much of this science began with Nicola Tesla and Dr Royal Rife over a century ago, Frequency technology is still an emerging field in health care. We are still very much in infancy with the clinical application of Frequency Medicine. But each year we gain greater access to new technologies which facilitate an understanding of how our bodies truly work.

Environmentalists, gardeners and nature-loving people will also enjoy this book because it shows how to help our great Mother Earth, to which we are intricately and invisibly intertwined.

My Story explains how I overcame advanced Lyme disease using a very different and emerging paradigm of health care and am living proof that it works.

Part One reveals the true secret of wellness, which is right in front of you.

You will be baffled to see how simple it is. You will be introduced to an invisible world of particles which are you in your physical form. You will gain an understanding of what your holographic body needs to stay healthy on a daily basis. You will be introduced to the technology developed by the brilliant minds of our era, and shown how this technology is going to add to our survival in modern times.

Following decades of scientific research and the development of highly tuned devices, finally we have arrived at the cusp of a new era in healthcare. Welcome to the exciting field of Frequency and Bioenergy (FAB) Medicine.

After reading Part Two, you will be able to take back your power and learn how to properly care for yourself, while understanding the importance of doing so. You will discover how cellular detoxification and vitality is the starting point for a strong immune system and perfect health.

It took a horrible disease and tens of thousands of pounds from my savings to keep me alive and force me to review my attitude towards looking after myself! Do not wait until it is too late. Explore what is possible and available for you right now. Frequency and Bioenergy healing protocols are helpful for many conditions besides Lyme, from allergies to chronic fatigue, parasitic burdens, fungal outbreaks and viruses.

Urgent Action Required

This book is written partly in answer to a call for action from the World Health Organization (WHO) to find alternatives to the antibiotic apocalypse about to erupt.

The WHO states, 'Without urgent action, we are heading for a post-antibiotic era in which common infections and minor injuries can once again kill.'

Herein lies one possible, replicable, financially viable solution.

Superbugs, Lyme disease and other chronic illnesses have become a major challenge to national health care systems and industries. Millions of people weakened by disease debilitates and demoralises the nation. A UK government report in 2014 listed almost one million employees who were on sick leave for a month or more each year. Sickness causes us to lose 130 million days per year, costing the national economy £100 billion per year. These figures are growing and are not limited to Great Britain alone.

Unwell individuals face financial repercussions due to high medical bills. Losing one's health and vitality also impacts one's emotional and psychological states, relationships and lifestyle. En masse we need to find creative solutions to these problems, learn how to stay well and change our attitude towards healthcare.

My wise grandfather had a favourite saying, 'Necessity is the mother of invention.'

The emergence of antibiotic-resistant superbugs and the global Lyme epidemic may just be that 'necessity'. We may not have any other option but to employ these emerging energy, light and vibrational techniques.

There is much here to assist those with daily health problems, chronic disease, and particularly Lyme Disease and its co-infections. My dream would be to see the majority of health practitioners and doctors incorporate these ideas into their clinical practices.

After reading this book, I hope you will be inspired to try this exciting path to wellness and encourage others to join you.

Through my associated website, www.pauletteagnew.com, you will have access to: up-to-date interviews with specialists, information on the proven devices that are used in Frequency and Bioenergy clinics, reading lists, research papers and suggestions for further exploration.

My Story

It's hard to know exactly when I contracted Lyme Disease as I have had many bites from bugs of all kinds and yet never had the red-bullet-ring rash or erythema migrans (EM). Most likely it was from a mosquito bite I received when working on the northern Kenyan/Southern Sudan border. I was working for a non-governmental organisation (NGOs) at the United Nations (UN) refugee and medical base. I trained Sudanese Catholic priests and nuns in simple trauma-healing techniques to help with the rehabilitation of child soldiers. It's hot there, very hot. The camps were low on water and we lived in single-skin wooden huts with chicken wire windows. Accommodation was basic, a simple bed with a territorial scorpion living underneath it and a surrounding mosquito net to keep out the zillions of flying bugs.

The sanitary conditions were very poor due to the lack of water and the used toilet paper went into open buckets for burning. We ate in an open-air restaurant with the food prepared and cooked outside. You know what flies are like; they take their pick of the fodder from kitchen to bathroom! At the same time, due to the Antonov shrapnel bombs, the huge medical tents were full of limbless men, women and children. Hygiene was a constant battle for all of us.

Under these conditions, it's easy to pick up a multitude of infections. As for bites, we had so many from everything that crawls, jumps or flies that no single bite stood out. People ask, 'Did you have a bite?'; gee, we were walking breakfasts for the masses. Prior to that trip, I had just come back from a great week-end break on the Kenya coast at Watamu beach in a friend's unusual treetop house. It also has no glass in the windows, allowing monkeys, snakes and mosquitoes to travel through the house. It's a malaria-rich area and of course we took pre-cautions. Our chef prepared fresh, vile tasting neem tea for us daily to ward off

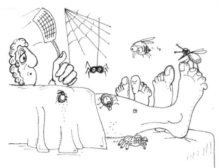

Dont' let the bed bugs bite!

the mosquitoes. Our stinky botanical body odour seemed to do the trick and I felt sure I had not contracted malaria.

Then halfway through the trauma-teaching programme I started to feel ill. I had no appetite, and developed a long list of symptoms; terrible fevers, chills, diarrhoea, headaches, digestive discomfort and more. Visiting the camp doctor, he tested me for malaria and concluded it was positive. He started injecting me with strong anti-malaria drugs. I was in no state to check or ask what was going on. This tipped my body over the edge.

Two nights later I found myself slipping in and out of conscious-ness. I'm not sure what state I was in, but I knew it wasn't good. Chris, my colleague, woke up to find me lying on the floor of his hut. He got up immediately, threw me over his shoulder and rushed me back to the clinic. The doctor found my blood pressure had dropped dangerously low and he spent all night pumping fluids into my body. I was flown out the next day for tests in Nairobi. After completing DNA tests, I discov-ered that he had misdiagnosed me. Nothing was found! No malaria, no tummy bugs, zilch!

As I look back now, I see now that this is when the Lyme disease started. I would discover later that many small insects and arachnids can infect you with Borrelia and its co-infections, not just ticks. This began a ten-year gradual decline in health as the Borrelia spread unknowingly through my body. It was worrying and confusing as repeated tests with doctors, hospitals and tropical medicine centres showed no infections, no reason for the endless barrage of complaints.

The slow decline as infection spread

As the disease moved through my body, organs and pathways, different symptoms appeared. Towards the end of that ten-year period, it became more difficult to think clearly and make decisions. I would walk to the kitchen and forget to make dinner, or leave the house and not lock the door. Booking a flight online was impossible. I was almost completely bedridden with fatigue and suffered regular five-day-long migraines. Heart problems, fainting and severe bouts of depression became part of daily life. My hand and feet joints became swollen and painful, and my knees started to collapse when walking downhill.

I was considered an attention-seeking hypochondriac, offered antidepressants, painkillers, and steroids which I refused to take. At night, lying on the bed, I would wake up with my arms and legs com-pletely numb. I would have to some-how flip myself over and force them to move. It was terrifying. Insomnia became the norm which caused me to turn to herbal remedies and on occasion pharma-ceutical sleeping tablets. After a whole week of trying to sleep with light bulbs flashing inside my head, I would give in and take a tablet to get five hours of rest. Pain would move around the body, mostly focussed in the muscles and joints. Some days there would be mini explosions of pain within the nerves of my limbs, spine and brain.

It was a confusing and demoralising time in my life and finally after ten years I ground to a halt, barely able to move, with brain fog and extensive body pain. I had numbness in my limbs and my left arm had become paralysed. I couldn't lift a fork to my mouth; things were very bad. This also led to a frozen shoulder due to immobility. My hair was falling out at this point and some days I would vomit for several hours.

A time for desperate measures

In desperation, a friend took me to see an acclaimed medical intuitive in Europe.

(What? Hang on before you park me in the loony asylum—think about it. At this point you would try and do anything, wouldn't you?).

As she 'looked' into my body, the first thing the intuitive said was, 'You poor thing, you have Borreliosis, Lyme Disease. The microbes are everywhere inside you, from feet to brain!'

Until then I'd never heard of it. She also mentioned a few kinds of parasites that she could 'see' lurking in the lungs, eyes and liver from various African and Indian trips. They were all easily treatable apart from the Lyme disease using her unique homeopathic approach. At last there was a name for my illness and reason for all the years of suffering. Research and potential healing could now begin.

After researching the many treatment options for Borrelia, I opted for a non-pharmaceutical approach to healing myself. This was in part because I have such a bad reaction to drugs, especially antibiotics, and also because I have always believed in a more naturopathic approach to cellular health and wellness. When you read Lyme patients' stories in books and online, they show that the antibiotic approach is not guaranteed to fully cure this disease. Large doses of antibiotics can cause more complications, weakening the body further. In addition to this, generally most doctors are not trained to support the body's detoxification pathways.

Successful treatment of serious conditions with pleomorphic and antibiotic-resistant microbes like Borrelia demand a different approach.

The use of strong drugs over months and years can cause serious side effects and weaken the body's immune system, gut and liver. My system was already badly weakened by ten years of disease and illness. What I felt I needed was something to strengthen my body and immune system—not batter it down further with strong pharmaceutical drugs. I'm also allergic to many Lyme and co-infection-preferred antibiotics (including metronidazole).

By this time, I was already in the final, critical, fourth stage of the disease, where the spirochete had penetrated the blood brain barrier and fully infested my central nervous system. This lead to the paralysis of one of my arms and facial palsy. By some grace, I had met an extraordinary practitioner who has been successfully treating Lyme and its co-infections for over twenty years. He has developed an approach to healing by uniquely combining Frequency technology and Bioenergy medicine. I immediately made an appointment and booked a flight to Europe where I stayed with friends who took me to the clinic three times a week. This was the beginning of my road to a full recovery. I have since met many people with Lyme Disease who moved over to Frequency and Bioenergy treatments after finding antibiotics ineffective.

To die or not to die? The battle begins.

It was a miracle. Prayers were answered. A solution had finally appeared. Although I was critically ill at this stage, my extraordinary therapist was determined to fight for my life. The battle had only just begun. Due to the advanced state of the disease, it was required that I be treated for many hours a day for a duration of four months. After those four months, my condition became stable and I slowly began to improve. I returned home where I continued to treat myself under the guidance of the practitioner. It would take another year and a half to fully recover, regain complete health and get back to a normal working life.

Battle—you might think that's a strange word for a peace activist and a yogi, but in the Bhagavad Gita, Arjuna the warrior (the indwelling soul of you and I) stands on the battlefield of life. This epic story is thousands of years old, yet perfectly describes our modern-day struggles and was certainly very relevant to my journey. It is said that the great warrior's knees were knocking and his hair stood on end, and when he saw the army spread out in front of him he dropped his bow and arrow and said to his charioteer (his Higher self) 'I will not fight.'

It was all too much for him. His 'enemy' was in fact all the parts of him and his life that did not serve him well, his weaknesses, his wrong associations, doubts and fears.

The ancient text goes on to explain that we need to fight these negative thoughts and attitudes. I also felt as though there was a battle raging within my body against the Borrelia, and that I had to conquer both it and any negative or unhealthy attitudes which would prevent healing. Faced with this massive struggle, I could have chosen to stop fighting—but I didn't.

When I began my treatment at the European clinic my extracellular Lyme count on the Bioresonance device was extremely high, almost at maximum infection. At that time, I was fully incapacitated. However, four months later I could manage to walk for forty-five minutes, compared to being immobile, and the nerves began to work again in my arm. My brain was relatively clear again and I was able to return to society as opposed to living a bedridden, pain-filled, forgetful existence. A year later my brain began to fully switch back on and I was back to teaching in my yoga school, walking five miles a day and laughing with life again.

Two years after starting treatment, I celebrated my return to life with a week of climbing in the Dolomites and enjoying eight-hour mountain hikes as high as 8500 feet; awesome! At last I was feeling whole in my body amongst the wonderful mountain air. Being over fifty years old after twelve years of disease-ridden hell and a chewed-up body…What a miracle!

Throughout this twelve-year battle, the Borrelia and co-infections had damaged quite a few organs and systems in my body, which took time and a daily home programme to completely rebuild. At this point, Lyme disease had fully taken over my life.

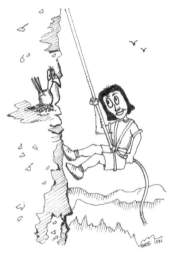

Cured at last.
Onwards and upwards!

Taking back responsibility

Okay, so how do you fight this microscopic enemy that has taken over your body and brain? For me it began by taking back responsibility and not giving up. There are days when you feel the benefits of treatments and other moments when you are knocked down by the Herxheimer reactions. These Herx's (flu-like symptoms) occur when your body gets overloaded while trying to detoxify and you feel absolutely terrible. Just remember during these moments that they will pass and you hold the power and keys to this battle. The Herx reaction is named after two doctors—Adolf Jarisch and Karl Herxheimer—who originally observed reactions in patients who were given mercury as a treatment for syphilis. They thought the reaction came from toxins released by the dying spirochetes.

Never hand your power over completely to any one therapist or doctor blindly. Question everything and do your own research. Lay out your strategy and your plan of action. Have your backup plans ready for the bad days and those times when you think you are getting nowhere fast. Always have faith in yourself and never underestimate your own strength, even when all hope seems lost. Where there's a will, there's a way.

A quick note at this point on the power of prayer, which in itself needs a chapter, if not a book of its own. During the days of darkness, when undergoing initial treatment and the battle seemed to be overwhelming, hundreds of friends worldwide held me in their prayers. On the second day of the prayer vigil, my practitioner uncovered a breakthrough with my illness. This was two weeks after starting the treatment with him. He figured out that he could break the hold this illness had on me. This was the day my life turned around and my body began to fight back. Slow and weak at first, but gradually with the enormous energy being poured into me globally and with months at the clinic, my body started to recover.

On the worst days, my friends assured me I would live and when you are in that huge black hole of doubt trying to find peace with the world, you need to have that reassurance. I feel so privileged to have such authentic, caring friends and family around me. Sometimes it's our nearest and dearest who hold onto us when we have nothing left. Facing the end of this existence—and coming back—changes you profoundly. Perhaps that's why I had to go on such a physical and spiritual journey.

This is my story, my chosen healing path, research and opinions. I am not a medical doctor and you must follow your own thoughts and pathway to health. Choose your own health practitioner and follow their advice. For all you wonderful doctors and therapists trying to help your patients fight chronic diseases like Lyme, I hope this book will give you some insights as to what other weapons you can add to your armoury. The ideas and concepts within may broaden your own research, treatment plans and strategies. For me, healing begins with an open mind, the willingness to try something new and the faith to go with your intuition and higher guidance.

PART 1

Frequency, Photos and Electrons
The Essence of Life

We are energy beings, made of photons and electrons, and
when aligned with the correct electromagnetic frequencies,
we exist in harmony and good health.

CHAPTER 1

Medicine of the Future– Frequency and Bioenergy (FAB)

"In every culture and in every medical tradition before ours, healing was accomplished by moving energy."

–Albert Szent-Gyorgyi, Nobel Laureate (1893-1986)

Frequency and Bioenergetic Medicine (FAB) is the term I have coined for the combination of technology and natural remedies. Later I will talk more about the technological devices which produce frequencies for healing and how they work. As there are so many phrases and names for different types of Frequency and Bioenergy medicine approaches, I will stick to the FAB acronym throughout this book.

Frequency and Bioenergetic Medicine (FAB) is the term I have coined for the combination of technology and natural remedies. Later I will talk more about the technological devices which produce frequencies for healing and how they work. As there are so many phrases and names for different types of Frequency and Bioenergy medicine approaches, I will stick to the FAB acronym throughout this book.

Increasingly, more and more people are fed up with the use of conventional medicine, its side effects and its often harmful treatment methods and medications. Nothing is worse than being constantly told: 'It's all in your mind.'

There is a reason people are seeking alternative and effective treatments; they want to be truly healed. Guidance on managing symptoms alone is not sufficient enough to eradicate an illness. They want to find effective solutions to permanently remove the cause of their health condition.

I believe that Frequency and Bioenergy medicine is the best means to treat and heal a wide variety of physical and emotional conditions. Awareness of the astounding healing ability of this combined approach will grow in the years to come. When this happens, the possibilities of healing will be limitless, causing a dramatic change in global healthcare.

We are gradually seeing growth in the number of doctors and practitioners moving away from treating isolated symptoms and towards an integrated approach. Many of these practices have their roots in natural forms of healing, such as the ancient medical systems of Ayurveda and acupuncture.

The rapid rise in complex, chronic diseases, exacerbated by poor lifestyle choices and environmental stresses, demands a comprehensive, contextual patient examination. This approach can be named many things by many therapists and may be a confusing labyrinth to navigate. Terms like 'holistic', 'functional' or 'integrative medicine' are used to encompass a wide variety of methods and techniques.

I use the term Frequency and Bioeneregy Medicine (FAB) as it includes the emerging field of light, energy, frequency technology and electromagnetic treatment possibilities.

FAB therapies are mutually inclusive, and usually have the best results when various techniques are employed together. It can also be used alongside pharmaceutical medicine. Doctors in Germany are already integrating various FAB methods into their clinics and day-to-day treatment protocols.

Most people today are 'programmed' to want an easy way out of their suffering by consuming a few tablets. Using the FAB approach often requires a change in lifestyle, diet and attitude. The collaboration of patient and practitioner is paramount to regaining complete wellness. In FAB medicine, a single device or technique usually is not able to fix everything. It normally demands the combination of a few techniques, tailored for each individual case. This may seem obvious to you, but if you are new to exploring healing methods beyond the allopathic model, it is an important concept to embrace.

When I was ill with Lyme along with its multiple co-infections my practitioner employed an array of devices and healing modalities together, creating a cohesive and powerful treatment plan.

Frequency and Bioenergy is not a new concept. For example, electromagnetic technology has been around for years and some hospitals already integrate this form of medicine. Orthopaedic Surgeons and Sports Medicine clinics around the world use specialist FAB devices, for example Pulsed Electromagnetic Field (PEMF) devices are found in many of the top football, basketball and baseball clubs.

Some of the well-known technology used in current medical practices include: X-rays, electroencephalograms (EEGs), ultrasound, transcutaneous electrical nerve stimulation (TENS) machines, electrocardiograms (ECGs), computerised tomography (CT) scans, and magnetic resonance imaging (MRI).

In time, we will begin to see some of the newer and lesser-known devices find their way into forward-thinking clinics bringing healing and balance. Some of these devices can also identify problems which were previously undetectable by conventional means.

Many clinics and hospitals still do not utilise FAB technology; however, this does not mean they cannot be found in smaller, private clinics near you. Some of this technology is now available at affordable prices for domestic use.

Frequency and energy

Throughout this book I will often use the word frequency which may require a brief explanation. Those of you who are familiar with concepts from physics and electrical engineering will know about this, but for those new to this world here is a brief summary.

In the pre-quantum world at the beginning of the 20th Century, it was understood that light and sound are examples of waves in space. As waves travel, energy is carried with them. The wave source is where the waves are produced, and they are detected when the waves impact on our retina, in the case of light, or on our ear drums, in the case of sound.

As a wave passes a particular point, we can measure the distance from one crest of a wave to the next. This is the wavelength of the wave. The frequency of the wave is counting how many crests of the wave pass the measuring point every second. Frequency is measured in hertz (Hz). Middle C on your piano has a sound frequency of 261.6Hz which means that just over 261 sound wave crests hit the ear every second.

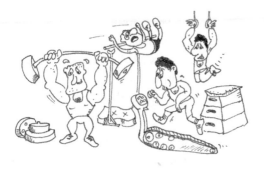

There are many ways to gain energy

The amplitude of the wave is the height of the wave, i.e. the difference between a gentle wave washing up on the shore, or a huge tidal wave crashing and destroying everything in its path.

If you reduce the wavelength of a wave, then more wave crests must pass the measuring point every second. So, as the wavelength gets smaller, the frequency gets larger. What is really important to understand is that the frequency is measuring how many times per second that a wave is impacting the surface it is hitting. So, the higher the frequency, the more energy is transmitted. This means that high-frequency sounds carry more energy than low-frequency ones for the same amplitude. Also, it means that blue light carries more energy than red light.

With the advent of quantum physics, it became clear that at an atomic level things are not so simple. It turns out waves for light and other atomic-sized particles have a particle nature and particles can behave like waves. So, light waves have a particle nature, particularly when they impact with matter. These particles are called photons. Each photon also has a frequency associated with it, so the frequency of a blue photon is much bigger than the frequency of a red photon.

All particles have a 'natural frequency', which is the frequency they will vibrate at when knocked. If you strike a molecule with photons with frequency equal to the natural frequency of the molecule in question, then the molecule will vibrate in sympathy, with bigger and bigger amplitudes.

The same principle is used every day in your microwave cooker, where microwaves with the same frequency as a water molecule transfer energy directly to the water and thus heat it up.

The resonance principle is used to transfer energy directly to destroy a virus, mould, bacteria and other harmful bugs; just by knowing its natural frequency.

These principles are the same as those used in Frequency devices and interventions. Similarly, there are 'energy' medical devices that use the same resonance principle to diagnose the state of energy in our body, or the presence of microbes or even abnormal cells.

Healers and their hands

Throughout the course of history there have always been people with the ability to heal through their hands. Many healers can remove blockages in the body which in turn enhances increased energy flow. Good healers are hard to find. They often become fatigued, especially when working with clients who carry the modern mind-set of, "fix me now—while I do nothing."

This problem stems from the expectations of a quick fix without putting in the hard work. This is a common mentality of today's generation, as we all live a fast-paced life where we have no time to be ill. People prefer to take a tablet so they can return back to their busy lives. However, the majority of chemical-based pharmaceuticals or "quick fixes" do not treat the root cause of the physical, mental and emotional problem. They moderate or alleviate the symptoms of pain and inflammation which does not benefit the patient in the long run. By getting to the core of the underlying cause, we can find a complete and permanent cure for chronic symptoms.

FAB therapies free blockages and increase energy flow through the body just as the hands of a healer do. When our bodies become energetically unblocked, we begin to truly heal. However, the responsibility for healing remains with the individual. It's up to each one of us to be responsible for our own health, and for this we need to understand why one has reached a point where the body can't function optimally.

Practitioners using Frequency and Bioenergy devices can help you identify the causes and contributory factors behind your illness.

With the help of your practitioner you will need to make a plan of action to reclaim your original strength and wellness.

The power of science and technology combined

"Though free to think and act, we are held together, like the stars in the firmament, with ties inseparable. These ties cannot be seen, but we can feel them."

—Nikola Tesla, engineer and inventor (1856-1943)

We may have messed up our nest—the earth—just as some of us may have messed up our bodies, but we have the intelligence to fix both. Daily breakthroughs are happening in science, biochemistry, computing and medicine. Particularly, the introduction of quantum mechanics has provided us wider understanding of the invisible world of energy, which I will examine later. Collectively these understandings are being brought together to create effective healing solutions.

Science and technology have come a long way with the help of many brilliant minds spear-heading the development of Frequency, light and energy devices. It's not a coincidence that they sit perfectly alongside holistic healing methods.

There are many FAB devices and tools available worldwide. FAB medicine encompasses anything that uses light, vibration, sound and electromagnetic energy. Frequency medicine devices can be used to detect, measure and treat conditions as they adjust electromagnetic energy in the body. Common forms are laser, infrared and ultrasound. Less common, but still very powerful are: electro-medicine, pulsed electromagnetic field therapy (PEMF), biofeedback and bioresonance devices.

There are also devices which work with the information field of the body. These devices use databases containing tens of thousands of pieces of information, which enable a thorough health scan, diagnosis and treatment. They can detect hidden problems within the body which may not be detected by conventional methods.

The cutting-edge world of FAB or 'electro-medicine' forms a whole new medical paradigm.

It has proven to bring many benefits, such as boosting hormones, reducing inflammation and pain, improving cellular vitality, production and repair and, as we will see later, enhancing cell membrane conductivity and transport.

These technologies are not intended to replace or diminish the role of our practitioners, rather they are intended to enhance the existing treatment protocols. There are already many practitioners in Europe using FAB technology with impressive and consistent results.

Frequency and Bioenergy medicine allows doctors and health practitioners to quickly and accurately gain information and insights into the patient's illness and causative factors. When you discover the ideal FAB combination of treatments you can often have a strong and immediate healing response.

Behind many illnesses lie hidden emotions such as anger, fear, and grief or traumatic memories. They can be buried very deep in our body/mind complex and may come to the surface during treatments. This is part of the healing process. In another section, we will explore how the "energetic" message of healing transforms into a biochemical one, thus creating the physiological response and vice versa. By triggering a physiological change at biochemical levels, we are able change the bioenergetic patterns and release entrapped "memories" at subtle vibrational levels.

Bioenergy medicine

The term bioenergy medicine can be used to encompass all the natural and energy-based therapies. This includes approaches which balance, unblock and increase the energy levels of the body, gene expression, the gut biome, organs and acupuncture meridians. They can also include, to name but a few: herbs, homeopathy, ozone treatment, oxygen therapies, vitamins and minerals, colloidal silver, sacro-cranial therapy, acupuncture, yoga, tai chi, live blood microscopy, salt caves, detoxification protocols and nutrition.

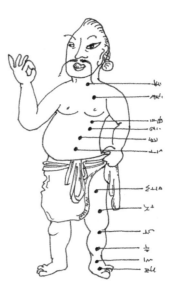

Bioenergy techniques work with the body

Lyme and other complex conditions tend to have a wide variety of ever-changing symptoms which appear as the disease progresses deeper into the body.

At each stage, you will be able to find the right FAB tool to treat and alleviate the many different symptoms including: pain, inflammation, insomnia, mood swings, anxiety or depression, chronic fatigue and even neurological disorders. Sometimes a treatment can be given purely to give you the energy to get through the day.

It's interesting to see that a century of significant medical advancement has led us back to the old ways of healing which have existed for thousands of years. In holistic medicine, the whole is greater than the sum of its parts, and putting ourselves back together becomes a very liberating and revealing journey. Ayurveda and Chinese medicine are all based on energy flow and have been around for more than 5,000 years. However, learning is never a closed loop—it's a spiral, and each time we circle back to a similar place in discovery, we are actually above it, expanding upward, very much like the helix of DNA.

> True healing is finding the deeply embedded cause behind an illness and using correct methods to heal it.

Getting out of balance may not be your fault

Originally, we inherited this earth in its perfection and lived in vibrational harmony, but in the last 100 years or so, we have, as a human race, screwed it up. Since the discovery of electricity, we have been using its power without truly understanding its effect on us and the planet. By setting up pylons and cables across our lands we have confused and weakened the magnetic fields of the earth and in our bodies. There are many cases of people who suffer from hypersensitivity to electronic devices.

Bees are also being affected by this, being unable to find their way back to their hives due to Wi-Fi and cell phone interference. We have built "global defence grids", which are affecting every aspect of the natural world. One can only imagine how they are affecting our own original, perfect vibrations.

Mankind has hammered out a few electromagnetic pulse (EMP) weapons and built the ground wave emergency network (GWEN) and then the high-frequency active auroral research program (HAARP)—unbalancing us at numerous levels. We live with mobile phones on our pillows and in our pockets. We have Wi-Fi blasting us day and night.

> We don't connect to the earth anymore, and most people live with some measure of geopathic stress (earth vibrations which have become distorted and harmful) in their homes, schools or workplaces.

Then there are the TV antennas and satellite signals, which track us every time we get on a plane. We get regular X-rays, ultra sounds; oh, and let's not forget the occasional nuclear fallout. It's just endless. Genetically modified (GMO) foods affect our DNA. These foods are not part of nature and can contain virus and bacteria DNA which can transfer to our own, or at the very least, transfer into the DNA of our gut flora.

With our own personal energetic defence grid out of alignment, along with the chronic toxic cellular overload, the rise of parasites, bugs, bacteria and viruses has become an inevitable reality. Our precious bodies are being infested with these unhealthy microbes, which are super keen to move in and reproduce in a weakened body. If you dropped your pet goldfish into a filthy tank full of toxins and irradiated dead water, how long do you think it would survive?

What message is this constant bombardment of "disturbing waves" giving our DNA electron clouds and biophotons?

Our DNA is trying to make perfect, harmonic symmetry and healthy bodies in every moment. The informational and vibrational harmonies in our bodies, minds, emotions and spirit are getting confused; and hence start producing sick cells, which can lead to weak immune systems and even cancer.

It's not too late; we can stand up and take our stance on bringing our bodies and world back into harmony. It's not an easy journey and we need to begin with healing ourselves.

It's ironic really—we build a massive defence grid against other nations, only to find we are destroying our personal shields and allowing the tiniest of enemies to kill us! We build a massive communication system—the internet—only to discover that it's destroying the beautiful communication system between our cells.

We rush to overuse and abuse the modern wonder drugs—antibiotics—which have a relatively short life span, while we ignore or ridicule the wonders of ancient medicines that have lasted for thousands of years and still work. Ironic or what? It's time to embrace a new paradigm.

I believe we are sitting on the verge of a new way for humanity; a time when our children and future generations will blossom through a blend of cutting-edge science and ancient modalities of energy healing and natural medicines.

CHAPTER 2

Photons—The Gift of Light

"The function of our entire metabolism is dependent on light."

–Fritz Albert Popp, biophysicist (born 1938)

As stated by many ancient writings, light is found at the beginning of all things. Thanks to the light from the sun, we have life on earth and the required energy for all things to exist. The fundamental particles of light are called photons; they take approximately eight minutes to travel from the sun to the earth where they reach our bodies. Photons not only carry energy relating to visible light frequencies (the seven colours of the rainbow), but they also carry the entire electromagnetic spectrum—gamma rays, infrared, X-rays, and even radio waves. We are literally living in a sea of photons where every living cell transmits and receives energy across the electromagnetic spectrum.

For those new to this aspect of science, in a nutshell, Photons are the fundamental particles of light. They have a unique property inasmuch as they are at the same time a particle and a wave. However, light particles are not the same as other elementary particles. Unlike other particles, physicists consider that photons have no mass. Also, although they have some characteristics of particles, such as angular momentum, their frequency is independent of the influence of mass. Neither do they carry a charge.

Phew! It's a lot to take in but what's key here is that in simple terms, Photons are the most visible portion of the electromagnetic spectrum.

There is an invisible and magical science happening around us—all because of these photons and their interaction with atoms. Everything in our universe is made of atoms: our bodies, the earth and the stars. Each atom contains a positively-charged nucleus (made of protons and neutrons) surrounded by a cloud of negatively-charged electrons. The energy that photons carry is responsible for the interactions between protons and electrons in the processes of maintaining life. As the photon strikes an atom, energy is transferred, which excites the electrons. It is this interaction that creates the energy by which plants transform carbon dioxide and water into 'chemical energy' or sugars.

The by-product of this miraculous plant activity is oxygen, the key ingredient required for our respiration. Hence the Greek word photosynthesis, phos (light) and synthesis (putting together).

> All of life, not just plants, is based around the absorption and emission of light. When light emissions and reactions happen within the bodies of animals, or plants, they are called "biophotons".

The Greek word bios means 'life,' hence biophotons are the photons of light within life itself.

Photons provide both energy and information

In 1923, Russian medical scientist Professor Alexander Gurvich discovered that the cells of all living things emit over 100,000 light impulses, or photons, per second. He called these impulses 'mitogenetic rays,' now known as biophotons. These emissions cannot be seen by the naked eye, but can be considered a non-material part of ourselves, connecting us to our outer world and environment. We are light beings, we thrive on light, every cell contains light, all biochemical reactions emit light and we heal with light. It is also important to mention that light carries information. Biophotons are often found in states of quantum coherence and can be measured with very sensitive equipment.

This area was widely researched in Europe and the US in the 1930s. More experimental and theoretical evidence was discovered by European scientists in the 1970s. It was in 1974 that German biophysicist and pioneer, Fritz-Albert Popp, proved the existence of biophotons, their origin from DNA and their laser-like nature (or coherence). He developed Biophoton Theory to explain the ways that biophotons control biochemical processes such as growth and differentiation.

Since 1992, the International Institute of Biophysics, based in Germany, has coordinated research into a field that promises rapid development in the next decade. Today, you can find thousands of papers written on biophotons.

> Popp said "Biophotons may well provide the necessary activation energy for triggering all biochemical reactions in a cell at the right time at the right place." This universal phenomenon of biological systems is responsible for information transfer within and between cells.

This assertion answers the crucial question of intra- and extra-cellular bio-communication, including the regulation of cellular metabolic activities, as well as growth, differentiation and even of evolutionary development. Popp also suggests that "Biophotons originate from an almost fully coherent field. In view of the permanent electromagnetic interaction of radiation and matter in the optically dense medium of a cell, it cannot be ruled out that an electromagnetic field of a surprisingly high degree of coherence may accumulate to such an extent that each molecule in the system is connected (or has the capacity to get connected) to every other one."

Popp explains how our molecules and cells use light for power and direction. For a biochemical reaction to take place, suitable activation energy for reaction components has to be provided by a photon (in the range of microwaves to ultraviolet). A photon of the appropriate activation energy is borrowed from the surrounding photon field to excite the reaction components and form a highly unstable transition state complex.

This transition state complex has weak partial bonds, which rapidly decay to allow the formation of a stable chemical product or products. Once the photon has excited the transition state complex, it returns to the photon field and is available for the next reaction. The average reaction time is approximately 10-9 seconds. Therefore, a single biophoton may be enough to trigger about 109 reactions per second, provided it is directed in a way that it delivers 'the right activation energy, as well as the right momentum at the right time to the right place."

> We are all light beings connected via an invisible field of energy.

Put simply, a photon emerges from the surrounding field of light and energy and returns once its job its done. Photons are the high-energy source that powers up electrons, making them ready for action. The highly-charged electrons then become available for multiple chemical and biochemical processes in the body.

Studies show that a healthy human cell emits more than 100,000 light impulses per second. Each chemical reaction depends on these light impulses.

> Every biophoton is an information package, a message on a very fine wavelength. Imagine a song being sung between molecules; harmonic equals healthy, discordant will cause disease (dis-ease).

If the information in the package is correct, then the resulting biochemical reaction will also be correct. If the information is wrong, the resulting reaction will be incorrect; leading eventually to an illness at the cellular level.

> If we do not change the message of the photons back to a healthy one, as new cells are made, they too will become disharmonious. We will literally become sick, one cell at a time.

In a nutshell, light is needed for electrons, ions, molecules, enzymes and hormones not only to function, but to function correctly! Truly, it is time to 'enlighten' ourselves and step into the 'light' for regeneration and wellness.

The holographic intelligent light body

Biophotons of light are also stored in our DNA. DNA continually gives and receives biophotons within the cell matrix. We have a web of light-connecting cells, tissues and organs within the body, which serves as an organism's main communication network. It looks as though DNA is acting under the control of biophotons, which, en masse, can be considered to be the body's holographic field and blueprint of information. Our 'biophoton information field' is literally directing operations at all levels, eventually creating the 'whole and perfect' human being.

This 'intelligent light body' is also considered to be the fabric of our interconnectedness with the environment, people and the world around us. What and who we surround ourselves with really matters. If we are unwell, it is important to live in a harmonious home, surrounded by loving and caring family and friends. We are truly connected with life in all forms; it is unfortunate that it is not obvious enough for many to perceive that consciously.

Neurologist Karl Pribram, along with many others, has postulated that the brain and nervous system's holographic biophoton field may also be the basis of memory and other consciousness phenomena. Overall, many of these discoveries have also provided scientific support for a number of alternative health treatments based on homeostasis (self-regulation) of the organism. These include somatic therapies like homeopathy and acupuncture. In traditional Chinese medicine, 'chi' may be related to our overall biophoton field. The Prana of Indian yoga physiology is increased through the practice of visualising light entering the body combined with well-known yogic movements such as the sun sequence and breathing exercises.

A healthy body is full of light.

Science is now showing what has been understood by holistic practitioners for many lifetimes—behind the majority of physical, emotional and mental problems, a causative disturbance is always found in the quality of biophoton emissions. Thus, when tackling any disease, such as Lyme, fibromyalgia and chronic disease, we need to address the illness at all levels, which includes light. It has been said that a disease and its symptoms are merely the means by which the body is trying to attract attention to the problem.

This is a very deep concept to master and, frankly, the majority of us are not evolved to a level of consciousness where we can heal a physical illness just by changing our thoughts. I believe this is what we know to be a 'miracle cure.' Ideally, we need to make sure we spend enough time in daylight, living in accordance to the sun solar rhythms (meaning going to bed at night!) and eating biophoton-filled foods; all of those things are crucial to total wellness.

The study and application of biophotonics (interaction between biology and photons) is an emerging understanding in science. There is currently a huge field of research taking place worldwide on many related aspects of light in the body. This research covers a wide range of applications: basic biological research, food quality control, cancer research, pharmacology, health prophylaxis, along with injury recovery and cellular regeneration.

There are just too many papers to reference here but a search of the internet will reveal a great deal of research has been and is being conducted in this emerging field.

The use of photon devices is an exciting development in many clinics around the world. Adding to the various treatment protocols, devices that measure the light emissions of a cell or tissue to reveal the state of the living organism are now available. For example, cancer cells and healthy cells of the same type can be differentiated by their biophoton emissions.

> Light-based technology is becoming one of the most powerful, non-invasive tools for investigating and healing life.

When we go outside and enjoy daylight (hopefully on a bright, sunny day), we absorb photons directly from the sun through our largest and fastest growing organ, the skin. However, between the modern, indoor lifestyles and reports to cover up and put sunscreen on, we are blocking light out. We should try to reverse this unhealthy trend by making time for our daily 'constitutional' and finding reasons to be out in the light. If you are in one of the countries where the Ozone layer (which filters damaging rays from the sun) has been depleted, you will be exposed to higher levels of ultraviolet radiation (UVR). Countries like Australia, Argentina, New Zealand and Chile are most at risk and residents need to be extra aware for the need to cover up more.

When ultra violet (UV) sunlight (photons) meet bare skin, our body begins to produce vitamin D3, crucial to our health and strong bones. Yet one of today's many lifestyle problems which is making us sick and exhausted is lack of light. In the UK, we are seeing a large increase in rickets in children. This is caused by a couple of factors. First of all, children and adults now spend most of their time indoors. Many hours are dedicated to school and work per day, breaks are often short and during them, we tend to use our tablets, computers and phones instead of spending time outside. Furthermore, commuting to and from work can take up to a few hours per day for many. Upon returning home, we are too tired to do anything but sit in front of more electronics instead of heading outside to play sports, work with nature or simply walk around the block.

The second problem which prevents us from filling ourselves with energy-packed photons is sunscreen.

> We are repeatedly told that the sun will give us skin cancer if we don't slap on a chemical-filled cream, when in fact we desperately need exposure to light.

It is very confusing with arguments in both camps so the key is to find a middle way. I choose to use a mineral-based protective sunscreen on my face when playing sports for hours outside, or on my body should I be exposed to a lot of sun on a beach for example.

Slap on factor photon—Sunshine vs. sunburn—the big dilemma

Let's put this in a sensible perspective. If you exercise or even sit for a cup of tea outside each day for fifteen, thirty or sixty minutes as the seasons change, your skin will adapt slowly and gently to the increasing strength of the sun toward summer. Of course, wear a hat and cover up in the midday sun and especially if you go on a sunny holiday.

Check your skin tone for simple guidance. Are you very white naturally? Have you sallow, olive or darker skin tones? The darker we are, the more sun we actually need and can also handle, as we have protective melanin already in place. But even darker-skinned people living a 'cover-up' lifestyle can burn if they suddenly head for the noonday sun. Monitor yourself; don't fry yourself by lathering your skin with oil at a beach. Hats are always a good choice to protect the crown of the head where hair may be thin and we want to prevent overexposure to the delicate skin on our faces (wrinkle prevention).

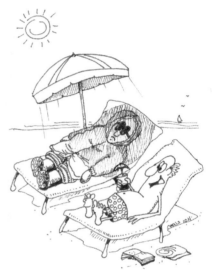

Now come on Dear, take your vitamin D

Humanity has managed to live naturally for tens of thousands of years, outdoors in daylight, without the need for sunscreen. A recent news report in Scotland stated that to prevent rickets we needed to take vitamin D tablets every day. The report should have recommended that you should get out and walk to the park or play football in the garden for thirty minutes, which is free, natural and healthy. Nor did it tell us to buy raw milk and use raw milk, yogurt, cheese, organic, free-range eggs, mushrooms, wild-caught salmon and other oily fish, as well as other products that contain essential vitamins and minerals, which all have the potential to prevent rickets. In summary: be practical, don't burn, avoid chemical products and get outside more.

Our unique light signature

You might say, 'I'm doing that, so why am I still sick?'. Well, we have to go back to what is disturbing the natural order of things.

> All forms of life, including human beings, possess a unique light signature. When outside signals disturb the integrity of this light signature, we start to see symptoms of disease in the body.

Anything from cell phone radiation, multiple vaccinations, bacteria and negative emotional energy can disturb our signature. These symptoms can be subtle at first and easily overlooked, but for as long as the disturbance remains, symptoms will grow in intensity until they can no longer be ignored. Uncorrected long-term accumulation can force millions of cells to literally live in the dark!

Not only physical, but also emotional and psychological traumas heavily influence the light in the body. If a trauma has not been properly dealt with, then the trauma remains a 'disturbance.' This disturbance creates a lowering of the energy and light in respective organ systems, a lowering of our gift of light.

CHAPTER 3

The Secret Power of Electrons

"Discovery consists of seeing what everybody has seen and thinking what nobody has thought."

–ALBERT SZENT-GYÖRGYI, NOBEL LAUREATE (1893-1986)

We are energy beings in constant vibration—made up of molecules (two or more chemically bonded atoms), ions (charged particles formed when a neutral atom loses or gains an electron) and the elementary units of atoms (such as positively charged protons and negatively charged electrons). This attractive pull of positively and negatively charged units is one of the keys to life on earth. Quantum physicists talk of electrons acting as both particles and waves.

In Jerry Tennant's book, Healing is Voltage (a good read for anyone interested in furthering their learning in this field), he proposes that an electron is actually a moving vortex of light; and, vice versa, light is a vortex of energy known as electrons. I have come to the same conclusion—light and its photon particles (in all frequencies) are vortexes of energy, and we are essentially vibrating beings of light! Our physical frame is like a hologram, a series of waves or frequencies of light. For the purposes of mechanical explanation and down-to-earth healing, let's look at electrons as we understand them according to current theories in chemistry.

When radiant energy from the sun (such as infrared and ultraviolet radiation), meets any substance—like water, a human body or even a metal wire—the energy is absorbed by molecules within that substance. This energy comes from photons, known as biophotons when inside the body. As a photon or biophoton strikes an atom, energy is transferred and may be sufficient force to cause the release of an electron. The flow of freed electrons between atoms is a small, but measurable, electrical current. The addition or removal of an electron creates negatively- or positively-charged ions. This interplay of ions and electrons creates the basis for most biochemical activities, such as the production of adenosine triphosphate (ATP) (which is essential for most cellular functions), enzymes, protein manufacture and detoxification pathways.

Electrons are the superheroes in the body.

A lack of bioelectricity is an indication of reduced chemical reaction in the cells of the body; hence, the body is working below its optimal level and we cannot experience wellness. Imagine our bodies as special vehicles made up of different engine parts (like the liver and nerves). These vehicles have trillions upon trillions of chemical engines, fuelled by electrons and photons. Every cell is like a mini sun, pumping out huge amounts of energy for its size, and all this power is fuelling the building, maintenance and repair of the body.

Therefore, no fuel equals:

- no action
- no movement
- no correct information
- no cellular communication
- no wellness

When we stop rushing and begin to look around, we see a world filled with life-force energy called Prana or Chi. The balancing and building of such energy has been the basis of healing in ancient medicines all over the world. From a modern scientific perspective, we may call this chi an unlimited sea of electrons and photons. The sun, sea, earth and photosynthesis of the great forests provides Prana or chi, oxygen, light and electrons. All of these are sources of higher vitality and health. Much of this book focuses on the necessity and healing power of the flow of electrons, originating from both nature and technological intervention.

The invisible world of electromagnetism

The earth herself is a huge, living matrix of flowing energy. It is plausible that the Ley-lines of old are conduits of electron flow in the Earth. When we go barefoot, electrons move up into our bodies, combating free radicals (more about these later) and recharging our cellular structures (this is true simply because the Earth is negatively charged and electrons will always flow from negative to positive).

The skin on our hands and feet are both good conductors, so getting your fingers deep into soil or holding a tree does indeed do you good. This is the essence of the new 'grounding' or 'earthing' movement and a reason to spend some time each day kicking off our modern, insulated, soled shoes and get grounded. Electrical currents are

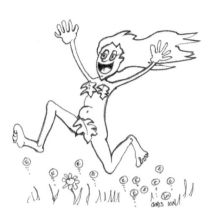

Barefoot is best for us

continuously flowing all around us. Electrons constantly move from a negatively-charged source to a positively-charged one just like in a magnet or down an electric wire. As this happens, a magnetic field is created. When the electrons are flowing with a direct current, the magnetic field is steady and can be measured some distance from the wire. The stronger the direct current, the further the magnetic field can be measured.

The earth has a North Pole and South Pole. The electric currents within the core of the Earth are so powerful that they create the Earth's magnetic field, which embraces the entire planet. This 'magnetosphere' shields us from harmful cosmic radiation and the solar wind. Many birds and animals have a 'magneto-sense' that helps them re-orient themselves and find their way, and it is quite conceivable that our bodies have evolved to make use of the magnetic field of the Earth, just as we need to make use of the Earth's abundant source of electrons.

We need the surrounding electric and magnetic fields and the low-frequency, electro-magnetic waves they generate in order to fuel ourselves, create optimum health and function properly in daily life.

However, in the past forty years, we have become bombarded by man-made electromagnetic fields from computers, Wi-Fi and mobile phone communication.

When we alter the natural, electromagnetic field around us, we alter our bodies. What we do to our environment, we do to ourselves.

The old English saying, "Don't mess up your nest", doesn't just refer to our own homes or throwing plastic in the seas; it also applies to the invisible world of electromagnetism.

> The challenge we face now as a human species is that many electromagnetic waves are not at frequencies that feed, heal and enhance our cells. Rather they disrupt and disturb their natural voltage and, if you like, also our "holographic" bodies.

I stress this point because we need to look at why we become sick and remove the multiple causes.

Electromagnetic and information fields can be measured all around our bodies. In every moment, these unnatural EM waves pulse within us, through us and around us. Given the chance, healthy waves will bring us back to our original, perfect harmony and balance.

> We are surrounded by a sea of infinite information, light, frequency and energy/life force/chi/Prana.

It exists within us and at the same time outside of the body. This information field carries its own intelligence. For example, it can instruct our bodies to make enzymes, produce urine or even make a baby.

Our bodies must have a means of transmitting information from one part to another which is essentially instantaneous and not limited by nerve conduction speeds or transport of neuropeptides. Candice Pert (Molecules of Emotion) discovered that reactions and biological communication in the body happen faster than what is possible through any other known means. The position of the electron clouds in the body is disrupted by trauma or harmful external factors such as e-smog. This creates a block or disturbance in our energy flow.

Exposure to singular, energy-disruptive events can be easily corrected by the collective 'holographic symphony' of a human energy field and bring itself back to perfect vibration. But, repeated over time, multiple disruptions lead to a scenario where our body can no longer cope with the imbalance.

The problem is that without this knowledge we keep making unwise, self-damaging activities and lifestyle choices.

We have lost the sensitivity to be in tune with ourselves and our environment.

Our bodies may complain about poor food choices, air-conditioned offices or being forced to sit and breathe poorly in a chair all day, but we just don't listen. We ignore all those subtle messages until we have become soggy, lumpy, stuck, degrading bundles of weak energy—commonly called a sick human being.

We moan about the pain and unhappiness without realising what we have done to our finely-tuned vehicle. Seriously, how long can the "orchestra" put up with the lead violinist being out of key, making a terrible noise?

CHAPTER 4

Energy Flow and Storage

Electron movement and storage underpins every activity in your 100 trillion cells and I'm going to explain how the body uses those electrons in biological activities. The biochemical processes of giving and receiving electrons are known as oxidation and reduction.

Electron movement—Oxidation and reduction

In simple language, when a molecule gains an electron or negative ion, this is called 'reduction'. When a molecule loses an electron or negative ion, it is called 'oxidation'. Oxidation is also known as rusting. For example, when an apple is cut open, it goes brown or rusts, so to speak. What happens in that process is that certain oxygen molecules in the air steal electrons from the apple cells, which then age and die. In the same way, free radicals in the body are out to steal electrons from healthy cells, enzymes and other processes, leaving the healthy cells and processes less effective or dysfunctional until eventually they get sick. If the cells continue to go without sufficient electrons, they will eventually die. Too many free radicals out to steal cause oxidative stress, which in some cases is considered the cause of autoimmune problems.

Although some oxidative activity occurs in the body naturally and for specific purposes, increasing these 'electron hungry' molecules through poor lifestyle choices can cause a severe imbalance.

The rise in oxidative stress, which causes ageing and increased acidity, can be brought on by the daily use of electrons without replacement, or by directly burning up this vital fuel for various detrimental activities already mentioned. This is part of the reason why the holistic approach to healing occasionally may not work. I've heard people say, "I get fresh air every day; why am I sick?" but they don't eat the right foods, never have bare feet on the earth, work for long hours in closed-off offices and sleep beside their mobile phones.

> Whichever way we get there, when our electron density is depleted, we enhance the oxidative process throughout the body.

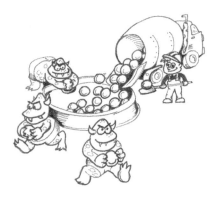

Free radical 'gremlins' steal electrons.

There are many things that exacerbate this oxidative process; for example, eating foods with trans fats, heavy metals, e-smog, pesticides and chemicals. Smoking, excessive alcohol and stress of every kind are also additional factors that can negatively influence that process. Oxidation and decreasing charge on cell membranes affects red blood cells (RBCs) as well as every cell in our body, including our immunity cells.

The opposite to oxidation (losing electrons) is reduction (gaining electrons or ions). Eating an orange, for example, which is full of natural vitamin C (an antioxidant) gives electrons to the body. Each time we are exposed to nature or an ionising device, we draw millions of negatively-charged electrons back into our bodies, giving our white blood cells the help they need to combat disease, invading bacteria, viruses and other pathogens.

Electrons also enhance the negative charge on the surface of red blood cells, which the red blood cells need to function as healthy, individual cells. Each and every one of us needs energy to move nutrients, oxygen, water and waste to and from locations in our body.

Energy storage—Mitochondria and ATP

Each cell needs a way to store energy and recreate it on demand, be it for DNA repair, an enzymatic reaction or to move a muscle.

Excited electrons are the basis of an electric current within the body. Through that behaviour, we create intracellular energy.

The simple science exposes again the fact that behind every biochemical/chemical reaction lies an electromagnetic process and wave of energy and information.

Everything requires energy. Like a light bulb or washing machine in your house, if there is no electrical current, the appliance doesn't work. Also, if the current is low, or if something is resisting the flow, it would generate a low-energy output.

As a biochemistry student at Manchester University, I was fascinated by the mitochondria, which are smaller organelles found within each cell. There are hundreds of mitochondria per cell, each manufacturing the molecule Adenosine Triphosphate (ATP). An ATP molecule stores photon-excited electrons, hence is responsible for producing the vast majority of energy in the body. When we have a good storage of ATP, we have high energy.

Mitochondria also need oxygen to produce ATP. With the correct oxygen supply to the mitochondria, they will go through an eight-stage biochemical process (Krebs Cycle) turning sugars, amino acids and fatty acids into energy stored as ATP.

The mitochondria will produce endless energy given sufficient, natural light, free electrons, oxygen, nutrients and water.

Are you now ready to scoot out for a brisk walk, eat a healthy snack and swop your coffee for fresh water?

When we need energy for a particular process, ATP is converted into Adenosine Diphosphate (ADP) whilst releasing its high-energy electrons. Mitochondria, the powerhouses of the cells, are fast becoming a buzz word in health and nutrition circles.

I love mountaineering and rock climbing, so I'm aware, as are most athletes, of the transition from oxygen-burning to anaerobic respiration after a hard workout. As we gasp for breath, we build up lactic acid and get cramps—not a good idea 150 feet up a cliff! Without enough oxygen, the ATP must use a different and less efficient process to make energy called the lactic acid cycle. It's a short-term emergency pathway that we use to keep us going and help us run away from danger.

The modern citizen can also reach this lactic acid build-up by living a static lifestyle that includes bad posture and inadequate breathing, as well as living and working in a poorly oxygenated environment. When our ATP is forced to work without enough oxygen, this build-up of lactic acid creates pain. At a cellular level, it increases that dreaded word: acidity. When the cells are acidic, we have fewer electrons, hence less power and less voltage.

Nobel Prize Laureate, Dr. Warburg, also discovered that cancer cells, bacteria and virus live and thrive in anaerobic, acidic conditions. Eating an alkaline diet has become a commonly discussed subject. The aim of this diet is to increase your electron count! The higher the alkalinity, the greater the electron potential in the food or drink.

Eating a processed diet, with a can of coke (pH 3-4) or drinking coffee all day (acidic), literally starves your body, not just of essential nutrients like vitamins, minerals and trace elements, but of electrons, or electricity—basically life-force!

Another way we store energy is via the transmembrane potential. This potential is the difference of voltage between the inside and outside of each cell wall. For an electric current to flow, there needs to be a difference in voltage between two points, A-B. This stored potential is measured as voltage. When electrons move and perform some kind of work, it is measured as amperage. We are all familiar with the batteries needed to run our gadgets, but inside our bodies there are trillions of cell batteries working for us day and night.

The presence of e-smog (electromagnetic pollution) will further decrease the cell membrane voltage and with it our energy. That lowered energy can take place in either the whole body (non-specific fatigue) or in one area, leading to a regional breakdown or illness in the cells and tissues. One example of this could be the rise in brain cancers, where people hold mobile or cordless phones close to their ears. Dr. Yakymenko told the New York Daily News "that using your phone for just 20 minutes a day for five years increases the risk of one type of brain tumour threefold, and using the phone an hour a day for four years upped the risk of some tumours three to five times."

My advice is to turn off the phone as often as possible, especially when you are in bed.

These transmembrane potentials were measured by Dr. Otto Warburg, who discovered that cells need to reside at around 70 millivolts for optimum health. Through natural occurrences, such as ageing, dehydration, toxicity, stress and so on, the transmembrane potential will drop.

When it gets down as low as 30-50 millivolts, we suffer from chronic illness and fatigue. Patients with cancer have transmembrane voltage levels of around 15-20 millivolts.

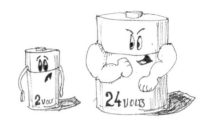

Much of the work of various devices in FAB medicine is aimed at increasing this cell voltage to help the body get more energy to heal. We are aiming to get back to this perfect cellular voltage by which we are supercharged and feel 'alive' deep down inside.

Supercharge your cell membranes and reach your 'potential'

The brain and nervous system are particularity prone to loss of electrical charge. Some of the conditions linked to a weakened cell voltage and transmembrane potential include:

- Heart arrhythmias
- Leaky gut
- Seizures
- Musculoskeletal problems
- Neurological conditions from a twitch to shakes
- Chronic fatigue
- Cancer

When we have the correct electromagnetic energy pulsing through our bodies, such as that created by a walk in a forest, we will also have increased electron density.

We are bathed and nourished by the earth's natural electromagnetic fields. Natural frequencies enhance the cell wall pumps to increase their activity, in turn enhancing the transport of goodness in and waste out.

We need to examine every aspect of energy production at a cellular level to consider how we get into these diseased and exhausted states.

Your thoughts, emotions, lifestyle and environment all contribute to your vitality and wellness. Ignoring one aspect will slow us down; ignoring many will make you sick.

There is only so much the body can take.

Connective tissue and the living matrix

Szent-Gyorgyi was an early, leading pioneer of the study of electrons and protons. His studies involved the protein collagen in connective tissue, which he found to be a semi-conductor, i.e. allowing the movement of electrons. He also discovered that the hydrogen shell (water) surrounding collagen also conducted protons. In essence, the water and molecules of the body are conducting energy (electricity) and information. This research was later developed by James Oschman Ph.D. of the Energy Medicine University. He explains the work of Szent-Gyorgyi and goes on to explain how the connective tissue (the most prolific substance in the whole body) is the matrix that sustains life by conducting electrons and their information from DNA to the outer reaches of the body.

Ground substance is the terminology used to describe the gel-like material filling all the spaces between cells, tissues and even organelles like mitochondria and DNA. It is electrically-charged and essentially reaches everywhere inside us, even the outer skin surface.

He called this 'The Living Matrix' and should we become 'damaged' in some way, (mentally, emotionally or physically) a blockage is created in the flow of the energy through this matrix.

Frequency devices and Bioenergy techniques are all tapping into this living matrix. They break down any energy blockages and increase the number of available electrons for maintenance and rejuvenation.

Studies suggest that if we are not grounded, or collecting radiant energy, the ground substance reservoir becomes low on electrons.

Bruce Lipton suggested that our DNA (and gene expression) is reprogrammed in response to the environment around it; this makes sense as an evolutionary tool. All species need to adapt to their external environment over generations, as well as surviving one lifetime. Food, temperature, stressors and danger levels, community involvement or isolation and so on have an effect on our DNA.

Signals from the exterior of the body and the input from all five senses send messages via electrons and photons in order for every cell to reprogram and survive. All our senses are collecting electromagnetic data from the world around us through sound, light, warmth, cold, flavours and scents. This collage of information propels our bodies towards repair, reproduction and replenishment. In every one of our cells, we have genes whose function it is to rewrite and adapt genes as necessary.

How we perceive our world is changing our genes and DNA. Hence, what we are thinking moment to moment is crucial for our overall wellbeing.

> A constant conversation is happening between our intelligent cells and our world.

Cell membranes lie at the interface of this vast communication network and I'll explore how to keep them super charged, healthy and operational later on.

I'd like to point out that hair is also an extension of our matrix and in older cultures long hair was considered an important part of both male and female strength. The story of Sampson and Delilah in the Bible may have a deeper message. Once his hair was cut off, Sampson lost his strength. I came across a fascinating story of native American Indians being used as scouts in the Vietnam War. When they had long hair, they could sense the enemy approaching, which allowed the troops to escape or prepare to fight. Once shaven, they lost this ability. Kirlian photography shows a larger aura of electromagnetic energy reaching much further beyond the brain when hair is long.

Regardless of whether these cases bear any truth, it does make sense that our hair is also conducting energy. We may yet find that hair, like skin, is actually very sensitive to various kinds of electromagnetic energy and able to absorb it directly into the brain and central nervous system.

> Massage, osteopathy and many hands-on healing therapists help stimulate a flow of energy and break down blockages in connective tissue.

From a psychological and emotional point of view, touch has even further healing benefits. All humans are hardwired to be held, loved and caressed. Pets are also great givers of attention and affection if you live alone. If you are too ill to look after one or travel too much, borrow one from a neighbour from time to time.

Free radicals and inflammation

When we have an infection, disease or malfunctioning cells, our body sends free radicals (also known as reactive oxygen species or oxidants) to destroy the diseased parts. These free radicals are out to steal electrons and, in a healthy, electron-rich body, will help our immune system destroy 'bad' cells. Phagocytes (neutrophils, macrophages, monocytes) release free radicals to destroy invading pathogenic microbes as part of the body's defence mechanism against disease. Inflammation occurs at a site of infection or damage where free radicals are active.

The body is super intelligent and to protect the rest of the body it will surround this immune battlefield with a vast army of electrons waiting for the infection and inflammation to die down. Once the fight is over, electrons will pour in and neutralise the free radicals before they can start breaking down good tissue.

If there are not enough electrons to do this, some of the free radicals will escape from that protected area and can start traveling to other parts of the body, prompting inflammation and oxidative stress, which, if left unchecked, can cause chronic disease over time. Hans Selye is a leading light in this area and has written much about the "walling off" of inflammatory pouches. His and the work of others, especially in dentistry, leads to our understanding of this "silent inflammation". For example, a root canal infection can lie hidden for decades, yet spill out free radicals and cause problems elsewhere.

Understanding the nature of free radicals and electrons is crucial for optimum health.

Nourishing yourself with electrons and enriched information photons enhances all healing pathways. The intelligent information field of your body will direct the electrons to infected or damaged areas.

Inducing this flow on a daily basis must be aided by efforts to ground yourself, spending time in nature, eating supercharged foods and drinking alkaline/ alkalised (electron-rich) water.

If your body has been reduced to a state of chronic or critical illness, simply changing your lifestyle may not be enough. Intervention with powerful Frequency and Bioenergy devices may be necessary to kick-start your energy healing process. Frequency and Bioenergy (FAB) devices are a technological miracle as they can compensate for the poor supply of photons and electrons caused by a modern lifestyle and toxic environments.

CHAPTER 5

What is Hidden in the Air?

There are a few key ingredients in any healing quest and alongside photons and electrons, negative ions are some of the key players. Many people have been researching the effects of ions for hundreds of years. More recently, Dr. Jaziri from the Rashid Hospital in Dubai described to me the many ways ions work, which brought about many "aha" moments for me.

From micro to macro, we are all essentially energy and informational beings. The structure of atoms means that a positively-charged proton nucleus is balanced by negatively-charged electrons. Positive and negative charges cancel each other out. Beyond photons and electrons, we move up to the formation of ions. Ions can be atoms or molecules that carry a charge.

Given the right conditions, all molecules strive to be in a state of perfect equilibrium. Vitality and harmony are our birthright, right down to the atomic level.

Electrons are 1,800 times lighter than protons and they can be easily dislodged from a molecule as they whizz around. When an ion gains one or more electrons, it becomes negatively-charged and is called an anion. Loss of electrons leads to positive ions or cations. That dislodgement process takes energy and occurs naturally both in matter and in the air. The air gets charged by the sun's rays, along with storms, waterfalls, ocean waves, lightning and some naturally-occurring, mild radioactivity from the soil and rocks.

Photosynthesis by plants also produces negative ions. Can you feel your energy and joy increase when walking through green mountains or a lush garden? Those negative ions are why sitting by a waterfall, a fountain or walking along the seashore makes us feel regenerated. It's also one of the reasons sanatoriums used to be built in the mountains or by the sea. In the old days, people may not have known about negative ions, but they did know that you got better faster in certain places. All metabolic activity depends on negative and positive ions joining and breaking apart.

Let's look at the healing power of negative ions in the air around us now.

You will have experienced, at some point, feeling better and more alive when in green places or perhaps after a big storm. The air is filled with a surplus of electrons held by negative ions, which, as we have seen, have a huge range of benefits.

A high density of negative ions in the air we breathe has been noted to: improve mental abilities and decrease depression, combat e-smog, increase vitality and help reduce bronchial problems.

As they clean the air from both pollution and bacteria/viruses (and much more), negative ions are released in burn wards to reduce pain, healing time and scarring.

Beware of that "positive ion" wind!

Weather patterns create ions as clouds rub together. That oppressive heavy feeling before a storm is caused by a build-up of positive ions, causing headaches and grumpy feelings! Lightning is a natural phenomenon that conveys the positive air ions to the negative earth during a storm and discharges them. This leaves us with a bright day filled with negative ions—the 'happy, invigorated' feeling ions!

Some people are more sensitive to weather ions than others and, as I research and write this section in Dubai, the Arabs talk of a wind called the Hamsin. It's hot and dry and picks up sand and dust as it travels across the desert. It makes you feel tired and lethargic, it can cause depression, anger, aggression and confusion. What's happening in the air is that dust and tiny particles like sand, smog or smoke attach to the negative ions and neutralise them, leaving the wind full of positive ions. This excess of positive ions can make you feel wiped out, agitated and grumpy! Some other famous positively-charged winds around the world are the chinook wind in Calgary, the Santa Ana winds in Southern California and the Foehn of central Europe.

Due to the way these winds form and travel, they are warm and dry with little water moisture. They cannot easily conduct electricity and hence discharge positive ions to the earth. People start to feel sick or angry, more accidents happen and wrong choices are made. If you live in one of these warm-wind belts and find your health, relationships and sanity suffering, get an ioniser or go on holiday during those weeks!

Take a spa at work

All the old healing spas in the world are usually high on a mountain or by the sea because we are bathed in a high density of negative air ions (and electrons from the earth) in those places. Compare this to modern life in a large city, which has little or no naturally-created negative ions, where windows are closed or sealed and the air is polluted, leading to an excess of positive ions. All of which can lead to high levels of physical, mental and emotional ill health.

> Air-conditioned offices and apartments are filled with energetically empty air. How can humans expect to thrive and be at their best when living in the poorest conditions?

However, some of the more enlightened companies are starting to add ionisers to their workspaces as they have been shown to reduce absenteeism and increase health, happiness and lead to higher productivity. A small investment for great return. Basically, if you don't have an ioniser at work or a city apartment, get one.

While in Dubai I was given a terrific, tiny book packed with years of research results on the benefits of negative ions. It's called *The Ion Effect* by Fred Soyka and Alan Edmonds and it's a must-have in your library. This little book came at just at the right time, and its bibliography is a treasure trove of research papers.

How many Negative Ions do we need?

The answer, it turns out, is quite a lot. Studies have shown that without this ionised air mixture, plants and animals wither and die. Various scientific statistics for healthy plant and animal growth show that around 1000-2000 ions per cubic centimetre of air occur in open, green fields. There is no known upper limit to the volume of negative ions which benefit humans. Concrete, glass and tarmac create dusty, dry spaces that use up the negative ions, leaving an unhealthy proportion of positive ones.

Looking at the statistics, we see that city air is reduced to about 300 negative ions and 500 positive ions per cubic centimetre. Inside a well-aired home in the countryside (no air-conditioning), there are about 800 negative ions and 1000 positive ions per cubic centimetre, and in a city office with air-conditioning, there are only 50 negative ions and 150 positive ions per cubic centimetre. We can see immediately that a life indoors in air-conditioned offices, homes and shopping centres is already creating a very unhealthy day-to-day existence for us.

Compare this with unadulterated nature and waterfalls as an example. The Needing National Forest Recreational Area in the Wulai township in Taipei has three separate waterfalls surrounded by forests and streams. It has 50,000 negative ions per cubic centimetre (the highest in all Taiwan) and one day resting there is said to relieve 120 days of accumulated fatigue! Niagara Falls in Canada, displaying the immense powers of water, is said to have double that: around 100,000 negative ions per cubic centimetre.

I grew up in Scottish mountains, which are full of energy, and everyone who has been to the Alps skiing knows how charged up you feel—despite being exhausted from four hours of downhill skiing!

Wherever you live, there are areas of natural beauty, parks, forests, mountains and seascapes. They will be filled with nourishing negative ions and electrons, just waiting for you to breathe and absorb—all for FREE.

Dr. Ahmed, who built his own ioniser for medical use, explains, 'At the higher natural concentrations, like 500,000, the body begins to heal.' However, he took this research a lot further and discovered that at 60,000,000 (60 million) negative ions per cubic centimetre incredible results occurred. He likens it to 'reformatting the body' and compared it to rebooting a crashed computer. His prototype JET gadgets produce these very high levels, showing extraordinary results in his clinic. He is seeing miraculous results on a daily basis. When I first met him in 2014, he had treated over 2,000 patients with no side effects or negative results. One case he discussed was a stroke patient who after three weeks of JET treatment in his day patient clinic was back to a full and normal active life; that is medically astonishing.

He also made another unique discovery, which I feel is of importance, but as yet we don't know why this happens. Out of the 2,000 patients who have been treated by this technology to date, those with O, B and A Rh positive blood groups reacted very quickly and with good results. Those with Rh negative blood groups took a lot longer and needed larger devices to get a similar result. He doesn't know why, so it poses a few questions for research yet to come.

CHAPTER 6

Supercharge Your Blood

Healthy red blood cells (RBCs) and white cell membranes are negatively charged and, as a result, gently push each other away. This keeps blood fluid, elastic, non-clustered and able to carry more oxygen to the narrowest parts of our tissues—in particular, areas of disease and damage. When they lose their negative charge, they coagulate and have difficulty reaching all the places they should. Another reason they clump together is to share electrons and maintain stability and health, but once they have their own negative charge again, they are free to break away to do their jobs efficiently. Given that almost a quarter of all the cells in the body are red blood cells, it's important to keep them happy and well-charged!

Cells can lose their negative charge by interacting with free radicals, those positively charged molecules looking for electrons to make themselves stable. Modern lifestyles lacking grounding and contact with negative ions can lead to our 100,000,000 cells trying to survive an onslaught of hungry free radicals, raiding multiple cell membranes for electrons. The result—chronic inflammation and disease.

To combat this cell membrane degeneration, our cells produce enzymatic and non-enzymatic electron-rich antioxidants. Their purpose is to neutralise the free radicals by donating electrons. Keeping fresh air pumping through our lungs is not just about oxygen; it's also about keeping enough negative ions flowing in to keep our RBCs freely moving and able to take nutrients through capillaries and hence into all the cells.

> Our lifestyle choices, environment, stresses and habits are undeniably part of the cause of our diseases and the reduction in our immune system's ability to fight bacteria and viral infections.

Dr. Krueger was one of the finest scientists in the field of negative ion research. In the early 70s he showed that even small amounts of these tiny particles could kill and remove from the air large quantities of bacteria, mould spores, colds, flus and similar airborne germs. It is believed that the negative ions attach to the bacteria

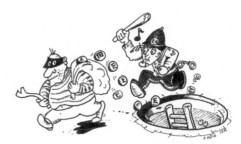

Find and eradicate the baddies

and form heavier clusters so they fall like dust. One particular study shows the decay rate of bacteria in natural air is only 23 percent per minute, while in air treated with positive ions it is 54 percent and with negative ions the decay is up to 78 percent per minute. Some hospitals now have ionisers in their intensive care and burn wards to help reduce infections. In short, the negative OH ions steal positive hydrogens from the surface proteins of the bugs, hence breaking them down with the by-product of this reaction being H_2O (water) molecules.

In an earlier study by Dr. Igho H. Kornblueh from 1958-1959, the use of negative ionisers on 187 patients showed that of those with negative ion treatment, 57.3 percent improved in all ways, versus 22.5 percent of the patients using drug treatment. The Nanzandoh Medical Clinic in Japan published results in 1975 from its research on negative ion therapy, finding it effective in the treatment of high blood pressure, gout, rheumatoid arthritis and tinnitus, as well as for various disorders of the nervous, respiratory and digestive systems, thyroid gland and skin. It was also found to speed recovery from illness and slow the ageing processes. Now that's something we all want! And it gets better. In another clinic near Ueyamada Hot Spring, in Shinshu Japan, they treated Alzheimer's patients with negative ion therapy and more than half were cured of the disease, recovering on their own with no further treatment.

Research into the benefits of negative ions started as early as the 1920s and 30s. Scientists around the world have been studying this natural antimicrobial and antibacterial healing pathway for a very long time. It's time to get serious, to help ourselves and transform our homes, workplaces, hospitals and our attitude. Let's prevent ill health by actively providing our bodies with one of the greatest gifts nature has to offer. It is all around us. Together we can help each other have access to free health treatments by protecting our wilderness and forest areas and keeping the seas and rivers clean! Nature is providing us with the means to stay well in many (mostly unseen) ways.

By saving our earth from toxicity, we in turn save ourselves.

The power of visualisation

We have seen that, at the photon level, transference of both information and energy are present. Electrons, our power source, behave as both waves and particles, transferring energy and information without physical contact. The meridian lines of energy connecting organs to the various systems also carry a current or flow of electrons/energy.

But for me, one of the greatest extrapolations we can make from all this science is to understand how and why visualisation and positive thought works (and it does). Often, we see and hear people talking about their beliefs and visualisations, where they see themselves being healthy or they imagine a health problem is dissolving away until its gone (e.g. a tumour).

How is this possible?

It appears quite simple, as we know that energy follows thought. The simple act of thinking 'wellness' sends a direct message to the body to be well. The healing power of photons and electrons is then directed to the area of our focus.

Much like satellite navigation telling us which road to take, energy and vibration is sent via electromagnetic information fields. Our thoughts and consciousness pinpoint an area that needs healing or requires an extra charged current flowing to it, and the body responds by doing so. Once that area is 'imagined', energy (electrons and photons) flows to it and the healing begins. The physical body is more tangible and easier to heal than say an emotional trauma or stored memory, but only because we are not trained to do so as children.

Once the 'energy' current is flowing back into the injured place in the body, the cells and mitochondria receive the power to speed up repair and rejuvenation work.

Often when cells are inflamed they become isolated and cut off from the streams of life force and information flowing though the body. Using mental imagery as a directional tool in self-healing is very valuable.

I've used visualisation all my life for succeeding at sports, where you visualise the activity done to perfection, building muscle strength by mentally going through the exercises. That same principle applies to healing.

The first time I learned to move energy was after spinal injuries in my late twenties. I could barely move my back and the burning pain was intense and relentless. It took courage and determination to enter the place of pain and imagine the vertebrae, nerves, discs and spinal cord being normal and well. Since then I've dedicated most of my life to teaching people how to rehabilitate their body, heart and minds and, at some point, inevitably we all have to go to the source of the pain. Bringing light, love and calmness to the pain or trauma and repeating this as often as you can throughout the day, or night if you're awake, leads to healing.

Complex issues like Borrelia, where the infection or chronic fatigue is widespread, require a more thorough holistic visualisation approach, but those suffering still benefit from the effort. In fact, everyone I met with Lyme who had a positive outlook got better more quickly and easily, regardless of the depth of their disease.

Everything is in motion and interconnected. Imagine our omnipresent consciousness and spirit directing and creating our physical existence by transmitting information through photons and electrons.

Emotions, like love, fear, anger or joy, are literally 'energy in motion', be it biochemical or electrical. They cause the movement of molecules and the release of hormones into our bloodstream. Choosing to live each day with happiness, passion and fulfilment is the basis of a healthy and dynamic life.

CHAPTER 7

Life's Great Miracle

Water is one of life's greatest miracles. We all understand that water is important for life, but do we know why? Water is known as the 'universal solvent' because more substances dissolve in it than in any other liquid. Let's find out more about water and what makes it such a good solvent and learn why it is a critical part of information transfer throughout the body.

One water molecule (H_2O) consists of two hydrogen atoms and one oxygen atom.

A hydrogen atom consists of a nucleus composed of one positive proton and one negative electron, which revolves around the nucleus.

Oxygen has eight protons in its nucleus with eight electrons revolving around it (usually drawn as four pairs of electrons).

Each hydrogen nucleus is bound to the oxygen atom by forming a covalent bond (i.e., by sharing a pair of electrons between them). That leaves six free outer protons in the oxygen atom. Because of the closeness of the electrons and the relatively large positive charge on the oxygen atom, the oxygen atom attracts more electrons than the hydrogen atoms. This leads to the oxygen side of the molecule being electronegative and the hydrogen side being electropositive, even though the net charge is neutral.

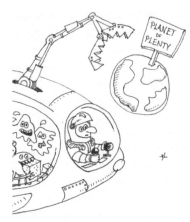

We inhabit a planet of plenty

I don't intend to overburden you with in-depth scientific explanations. However, I do believe that by knowing the chemistry within your body, you will gain an appreciation of your marvellous inner makeup and use it to your advantage.

The type of arrangement above makes water a 'polar' molecule. The positive region of a H_2O molecule is attracted to the negative region of another and weak hydrogen bonds are formed. Joining, stretching, bending and breaking the hydrogen bonds leads to the formation of water molecules and H+ and OH- ions, which react together to form water again. One hydrogen atom, although covalently attached to one oxygen atom, will draw another oxygen atom toward it and so on. We could imagine long chains of water molecules, but, in reality, it would be more like three-dimensional clusters.

Water molecules are constantly vying with each other for their shared electrons. It is the polarity of water molecules that attracts other substances and, in numerous cases, the attraction is strong enough to break the bonds in other molecules, allowing them to dissolve. The weak H_2O bonds are part of life's miracle, with molecules being broken down and reassembled on a continuous basis.

The fluidity created by the giving and taking of electrons is key to the chemical reactions necessary for life on earth.

With water being the 'universal solvent', we need an abundant, clean supply of water to drink and, without it, nothing works. Later I will explain more about the benefits of water in our bodies, but for now, did you know that babies consist of approximately 78 percent water, dropping to about 60 percent after one year? Adult men are roughly 60 percent water and women 55 percent, which is lower because they have more fat cells. Muscle tissue contains 75 percent water and fat 45 percent. The more fat you carry, the less hydrated you are which adds the additional problem of obesity.

Mae-Wan Ho, author of Living Rainbow H_2O and biophysicist, explains clearly how water is critical to all activities in the body. She explains, 'The liquid crystalline structure of organisms depends essentially on the liquid crystalline water that aligns itself along the enormous amount of interfaces. It is excited water that is easily split by infrared photons absorbed in photosynthesis, into protons, electrons and oxygen. The protons and electrons are positive and negative electricity that basically power molecular machines, which because of the water associated with them can transfer and transform energy at close to 100% efficiency. The pervasive liquid crystalline water also enables the molecules to act in a highly-coordinated way, approaching quantum coherence.'

She goes on to say, 'only quantum coherent proton and electron transport can account for the instantaneous or faster than light intercommunication that enables distant neurons to fire together, which is not different from distant muscle fibres acting together in a perfectly coordinated way... This enables ultimately each individual molecule to intercommunicate with every other, and water holds the key to the intercommunication, as well as memory of the macroscopic wave function that characterises the individual organism.'

Quite simply, without correct hydration, we simply cannot function at our best in any way. Do you drink enough fresh water every day? Is it the right kind of water?

The fourth phase of water

One of my all-time favourite books is The Fourth Phase of Water by Gerald H. Pollack. This book has me totally entranced. His scientific explanations and new paradigms are enlightening and challenge the existing model explaining particles and energy. In it he states that only internal energy is needed to cause particles to move ceaselessly. He shows how Brownian motion—also called Brownian movement—and other associated theories are not the only factor in the equation of atomic movement or activity.

Radiant energy from external sources such as the sun and earth are continually energising water particles and molecules.

He proposes that electromagnetic energy from sources such as the sun and the earth power up these Brownian motions.

Experiments show that the most effective and relevant wavelengths that give energy lie in the infrared range. Warm water, due to its atomic structure, radiates significant amounts of infrared energy. From this knowledge, we can start to see why infrared devices, like saunas and mats (to lie on), are so supportive during the healing journey and part of FAB treatment protocols.

In addition to solid, liquid and vapour, gas and plasma states, Pollack explains the existence of an 'ordered' or what he calls the 'fourth phase' of water. This particular phase forms next to a flat or spherical hydrophilic surface (i.e., one with a strong affinity for water), such as a gel, polymer, biological surface or monolayer. This structured type of water essentially builds an exclusion zone (EZ) next to the hydrophilic surface, which keeps solutes out and it is therefore known as EZ water (or H_3O_2). Unlike bulk water, EZ water is highly negatively charged. The structure of EZ water is created when incident light is shone on the water.

Infrared energy is absorbed by water, which separates the H2O molecules. The negatively-charged parts (OH-) become the EZ and the positive parts form hydronium ions (H_3O+), which disperse through the "bulk" water. The more light that is added, the more the separation of charge occurs. As the EZ layers build, they create a honeycomb lattice (containing six oxygen and six hydrogen atoms)— similar in fact to the structure of ice. It is the increased ratio of oxygen to hydrogen (when compared with bulk water) which causes the negative charge of EZ water.

Light induces the splitting of water, separation of charge and the generation of EZ water, which influences the movement of particles.

This difference in charge is vital to all life.

The charge creates energy, which can be released from water in many ways as electromagnetic, physiochemical, electrical and mechanical energy.

Hydrophilic particles suspended in water will be surrounded by a negatively-charged EZ layer, which in turn is surrounded by positive particles. When more than one EZ-surrounded particle is present, the particles become attracted to each other and move towards the highest positive charge (which will be strongest between them). In his experiments, Pollack has shown how a beam of light (photons) shone through water causes its colloidal particles to draw closer together. The microspheres within the water move toward the light, concentrating around it.

Biophysicists have also used the energy from light to move and trap particles with an experimental tool known as optical tweezers. As light passes through particles it refracts, causing its momentum to change. As the photons lose momentum, the particles gain that energy and this can be used to manipulate them. Using optical tweezers, light from a laser beam is used to trap particles at the region with the highest intensity. Experiments using optical tweezers have been used to show the force within EZs, which may potentially influence cellular activities.

Pollack's research suggests that light induces the splitting of water, separation of charge and the generation of EZ water, which influences the movement of particles. This difference in charge is vital to all life. It has even been proposed that water droplets in our atmosphere are composed of negatively charged EZ outer 'shells', whereas the inside is composed of hydronium ions.

All charged entities (such as membranes, proteins and DNA) interface with water to create EZs, which in turn bear charge, meaning they carry electrical potential. This charge creates energy, which can be released from water in many ways as electromagnetic, physiochemical, electrical and mechanical energy.

Water can convert energy into light.

Electromagnetic energy is the same as light or heat. An experiment with salt water in a test tube demonstrated that when exposed to microwaves or a radio frequency signal, the water catches fire—light and heat! Physiochemical energy stored between the bonds in water molecules is transformed when those bonds form or break.

Electrical energy is important for cellular activity, as the movement of electrons is necessary for voltage to work. Differences in the electrical potential exist between the interior and exterior of cells and we know that water conducts and retains electrical energy.

This energy then becomes mechanical in nature and can be observed as cellular activity, moving molecules to build, repair and heal the body.

Stated very simply, without correct hydration the body will not be able to make enough energy and do its work correctly.

Interestingly, self-driven flow of water has been observed in submerged horizontal tubes, perhaps due to interactions between water molecules and the hydrophilic surface of the tube. The flow became faster under incident light—perhaps this was due to the formation of EZ water. It would be interesting to see how the effect of light enhances blood flow through tight capillaries in the human body.

Creating new DNA

French scientist and immunologist Jaques Benveniste first discovered that water has memory by successively diluting a biologically active substance until only water remained. This is similar in fact to the making of homeopathic remedies. What Benveniste found was that when he later poured the serially diluted water onto cells, it would trigger the same molecular dance as the actual original substance. Due to difficulties in reproducing the results, he was ridiculed and this research was put aside until Nobel laureate Luc Montagnier carried on his work to show that indeed water does carry and transmit information.

A mind-blowing experiment by Montagnier shows how light transmits information as well as giving energy. Imagine two sealed and separated test tubes. Tube A filled with water containing DNA. Tube B filled with pure water. Both tubes were placed beside each other and exposed to electromagnetic energy.

Later, the water from tube B was poured into a solution containing the raw materials for DNA and new DNA strands grew. This could only be possible if Tube B water carried the structural information to do this.

Clearly the information was exchanged via electromagnetic or 'photon' transmission from one flask to the other and then the biophotons knew how to use the raw ingredients to create the new DNA.

Biophotons are carrying vital information through our water-based structures.

Science and cutting-edge discoveries are now able to explain why therapeutic interventions using light and electromagnetic energy devices are healing our bodies. Imagine a laser beam shining through your body to an affected area, carrying energy information and electrons for healing. Many FAB laser and biophoton devices use this concept and carry healing information into our cells and molecules.

As well as light and healthy electromagnetic frequencies, we require a suitable amount of clean and natural water in our bodies to maintain health—from molecular to gross levels. Being 'toxic' and bombarded by destructive electromagnetic frequencies directly opposes us being well, maintaining homeostasis and having correct cellular voltage.

CHAPTER 8

Water Can Heal

Bodies require a helping hand to stay in balance during intense detoxification and deep healing programmes. It is also hard to maintain the perfect homeostasis on a day-to-day basis when we are living with air, food and water pollutants and inadequate cellular nutrition. I arrived at a point when the symptoms of my chronic and advanced Lyme were extremely uncomfortable: five-day migraines, six-hour vomiting sessions, arthritis in most of my joints and constant pain throughout my body.

A lovely friend brought me some alkalised, ionised water, which she suggested could help. Quite frankly, at this point you would try anything, and I dutifully gulped back about two litres during her visit. The migraine stopped within a few hours and the next morning my joints were no longer swollen and painful. What would you do then? Try more of course, and she drove an hour every three days to supply me with this water.

I'm not saying ionised water can cure Lyme or any other disease, but it did help relieve many of the symptoms. I was hooked and decided to take the plunge and get my own water ioniser. It has been one of the best investments for my health ever. If there was ever a fire in the house, I'd grab my passport, wallet and ionising water machine!

As a keen mountaineer and sports enthusiast, drinking water was already high on my agenda. I've also tried many kinds of filters during my travels to Third World countries for adventures and work. In places like Africa and India, you want to ensure giardia and other waterborne bacteria are filtered out. Here in the western world, we need to filter out chlorine, fluoride and all the other chemicals that are added to tap water to make it 'safe'.

Having spent a great deal on various water machines, I've settled with the one that actually works (visit www.pauletteagnew.com for details). Note that there is a difference between alkaline water and electrically-produced alkalised water. Alkalised is the only system that is stable enough to produce high quality antioxidant water and it must be freshly made, not bottled and stored. Compare 'active' water from a racing, high, mountain stream bouncing down the hills to 'inactive' water sitting in a pond at the bottom. The electrical process is akin to a lightning strike, which naturally alkalizes or ionizes water in the wild.

We are made of water

Correctly hydrating our cells is absolutely crucial to the healing journey. When we fully appreciate all the roles of water in our lives, we look at a glass of water differently! As we age, we carry less water in our bodies, which is easily seen in the loss of height as the intervertebral disks lose their plumpness.

> While we are on the benefits of correct hydration, did you know that keeping youthful skin is mostly about cellular hydration rather than applying expensive face creams?

Before we go nuts and overhydrate, any doctor will tell you the average intake is about two litres a day. Obviously, larger bodies, a hot day, or running around a football pitch will all use up more, so find your correct intake and use it as a rough guide. Most people think their tea, coffee and sodas are part of the two litres, but, in fact, it's the opposite; those drinks cause us to lose water as they are diuretic and the sugar in those drinks requires water molecules to be metabolised.

The average adult body is comprised of around 75 percent fluids and 25 percent solids (a similar proportion of our planet's water to earth ratio), but brain tissue has a higher percentage of fluid at around 85 percent water. Due to our built-in survival mechanisms, if we don't hydrate properly, water will be taken away from less important areas like our skin, and given to those that truly need it, like the brain. Let's face it, if you can't think properly you won't be able to escape the tiger or plan how to get food and shelter for your tribe. Brain cells also contain and demand higher oil content than anywhere else in the body. Our ingenious bodies will take the most important building blocks for health and use them first in the brain.

One great exponent of hydration is Dr F. Batmanghelidj. He is one of the world's leading specialists in this field, and his seminal book, Your Body's Many Cries for Water, is a fantastic read. I read it about fifteen years ago and have been quoting him in all my lectures ever since. This work is a classic based on hard evidence and years of research. He discovered that water could cure a majority of illnesses while being imprisoned for nearly three years in an Iranian jail.

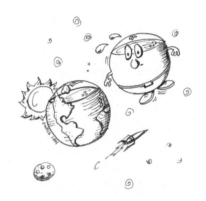

We are water babies

As a doctor, all he could give fellow sufferers was water, and many of their diseases miraculously healed. After regaining his freedom, he carried on this research and has shown how a multitude of diseases and conditions can be remedied or reversed by correct hydration. This includes ulcers, digestive inflammation and pain, rheumatoid arthritis, high blood pressure, excess weight, stress, asthma, back pain, migraines, hangovers, allergies and depression—to name just a few. In addition, water helps regulate body temperature by absorbing heat generated by your metabolism and eliminating excess heat through sweating. It is essential for the digestion of food, lubricates your joints and fills your spinal disks.

Are you convinced?

The concept Dr Batmanghelidj puts forward is that conventional medicine and science follow the old paradigm that the solute (the molecules) is the driving force or reactive regulator and active ingredient in all the body's functions, whereas he believes it is actually the water molecules (the solution). This is shown over and over again with water being a living medium of communication and exchange, as well as a reservoir of energy. In a nutshell, the biochemistry of life is based on water.

As we have seen in previous sections, water is both the basis of all metabolic reactions and electron transfers and serves as a carrier of information. Remember the DNA transfer experiment where information, via the electromagnetic current, was transferred into water, which then passed on that message to a solute to create new DNA?

> Good water and correct hydration are crucial to cellular
> health, rejuvenation, anti-ageing, detoxification, electron or
> electric current charge, healthy blood flow and so much more.

Living crystal water babies

Water has been shown to be restructured by various kinds of energies and magnetic fields. The work of Dr Masaru Emoto shows how water changes according to the energies around it, like music, prayer or intention. He showed this by freezing the water and then photographing its structure. Happy, healthy vibrations would create beautiful crystalline structures, whereas aggression and negativity created discordant patterns. This helps explain how carrying negative thoughts about yourself and your world, or being surrounded by negative or aggressive people, affects your health at cellular level.

This research, and more, leads us to a simple conclusion.

> Given that we are predominantly water, and because water
> alters according to its environment, it's up to us to direct and
> determine what kind of water lies inside of us. This in turn
> will influence what kinds of bodies and minds we all have.

If we surround ourselves with positive and beautiful vibrations, as well as spending time in nature, we should be healthy! We are essentially a living, liquid, crystal being. We are mirrors of the energy inside and outside of us.

Every cell is a radio transmitter and receiver of frequency and vibration. Unfortunately, life is usually quite different than the ideal for most people. Let's face it, most people don't have a high level of emotional happiness, equanimity or spiritual oneness. Humans tend to carry some kind of negativity such as past pain, fears, worry, stress, anger and insecurity. Without knowing it, these are constantly charging and programming water molecules in your body with that frequency minute by minute. A word of warning: the toxic, irradiated, dead molecules (junk food and microwaved dinners) contain water molecules which carry a less than healthy message into our cells.

Working and sleeping in disturbed electromagnetic fields for hours on end, having little access to a fresh supply of negative ions and e-smog bombardment are all changing our living, liquid-crystal, water-based bodies. No wonder they start to complain and eventually function at less than optimum.

One of the solutions to this less-than-optimal situation is to keep a fresh and powerful supply of water streaming through our bodies in order to change and refresh the water in every cell each day. That way, even though we are contaminating the body in many other ways, it still has the opportunity to eliminate unwanted waste and old vibrations!

On the subject of hydration, I read a story years ago about a surgeon doing an autopsy on a middle-aged man who died of a heart attack. The man who died was very successful

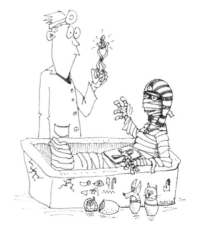

I think that is mine

and wealthy, but extremely stressed most of the time. When they opened him up, the surgeon said that his heart looked like a dried date. His organs looked cooked and dehydrated.

> Stress is drying you up, whether it is from an illness, worry, trauma, e-smog or another cause.

Stress also creates free radicals. These in turn attack the cells and artery linings and disrupt many essential biochemical functions. In response, the body produces cholesterol to neutralise the free radicals and repair cell membranes, both with the crucial phospholipids (fats) and also via the electron clouds carried in healthy fats. Please note this is not the ingested "cooked, hydrogenised or pasteurised" fats found in processed food. Good cholesterol integrates with the cell membranes to help stop water loss from the cells. Too much cholesterol because of chronic stress leads to cellular dehydration and malnutrition because it coats the cells like cellophane wrapping. Fresh water and nutrients can't get in and waste can't get out.

CHAPTER 9

Alkalised Water—
The Best Antioxidant

We need to choose water that has high anti-oxidant potential (to refresh our memories, this means water that carries a high proportion of negative ions to be given away). From other sections of this book, we see that ions are crucial to cellular wellness and therefore whole-body health. The Oxidation Reduction Potential or Redox Potential (ORP) of fluids can be measured; you are looking for water with about -300 to -800 ORP. These water molecules are great donors of electrons and, when consumed daily, can aid our bodies in their healing and "energy generation" functions. In comparison, bottled water has a high positive ORP and will actually steal electrons, causing you to lose energy and creating more problems.

Free radicals are the current buzzword and the sale of antioxidants has become big business. Remember free radicals, also known as oxidants, are out to steal electrons. Antioxidants are donors of electrons, so when you go out to buy 'antioxidants' you are actually buying a store of spare electrons. The common ones are glutathione, vitamin C, beta-carotene, vitamin E and superoxide dismutase (SOD). They give away electrons by oxidising themselves, but the remaining molecule is stable enough to not become a free radical.

> Drinking ionised, alkalised water, with its abundant supply of electrons, will go a long way toward neutralising the sea of free radicals in our bodies.

Ionised water is created by passing filtered tap water over electrically-charged plates, increasing the reductive potential. Tap water by itself may have an average oxidative potential of around +300, which will go into your body and steal electrons to neutralise it. Many doctors now suggest that alkalised water should be part of any healthy lifestyle. Dr William Kelly, author of Cancer Cure says, "Alkalised water produced by a water ioniser has become the most important advancement in health and a stunning one, at that." Using good water, like many of the points discussed in this book, aims to normalise or balance our cellular mechanism as we go about our everyday life.

The higher the alkalinity or pH of the water, the more negatively-charged ions are available as donors to the body. The lower the pH, i.e., acidity, the more positively-charged the water. The positively-charged water also has many benefits, but not for drinking.

Good hydration is crucial to the proton pump in the cell membrane, which pulls hydrogen (H+) molecules through to the outside of the cells. This builds up a positive charge, which is then attracted back into the cells. As the H+ is drawn through the membrane, ATP is produced for the cells to use for energy.

Water is one of the greatest donors of H+ in the body. When we decrease our water intake, we automatically reduce the H+ needed to produce molecules of ATP and thus diminish our supply of cellular energy. Everything in our bodies is designed to perfectly make energy, heal, reproduce and regenerate. We have to wise up and give our body the right tools and ingredients. Stop harassing it with bad decisions (most of which are just habits)!

Lack of water = Lack of energy

Let me share another small point on energy production and conservation. When we're sick, we don't want to waste precious life force by drinking water that contains toxins. This puts a huge strain on the same cells and organs that are fighting the bugs. Drink good, filtered water.

Running water makes more sense

When water sits in pipes, tanks and bottles all day, the H2O molecules gradually become more clustered together. These larger 'bundles' have to be broken down and restructured to enable the individual H2O molecules to be used. This takes energy, and if your body is sick, you are asking more of an already burdened energy system.

Bottled water is most often slightly acidic (an oxidant) and an electron stealer. When we lived in a toxin free world, with the earth's magnetic fields intact, we were drinking fresh spring water and it would have been full of minerals and rich in negative ions. How many of us live in such a place now? Think about your water supply. Does it come from reservoirs? Has it sat in tanks and travelled miles in metal or plastic pipes in straight lines? How many chemicals have been added to make it 'safe'? What vibrations, magnetics and geopathic stresses has it been subjected to? Has it been recycled a number of times from sewerage? Is it desalinated?

The answer to one or more of those questions is probably yes. This is why our 'natural tap water' is not natural and does not have enough free electrons to maintain super healthy bodies. Offices and workplaces that care about their staff could supply ionised water to keep brains active, increase productivity, combat stress, enhance staff well-being and reduce sickness absenteeism.

Drinking ionised, alkalised water, with its abundant supply of electrons, will go a long way toward neutralising the sea of free radicals in our bodies and enhancing overall well-being.

In forward-thinking, Japanese hospitals, the medical teams and hospital workers are allowed free access to ionised water. Japan is very much leading the way with doctors using ionised water of various pH levels to treat many conditions and even kill germs. From dressing burns to curing gangrene, ionised water is effective. Water at pH 2.5 kills bacteria, including methicillin-resistant staphylococcus aureus (MRSA)! Meanwhile in the US, Dr Gabriel Cousens, author of Conscious Eating, says it simply: 'Water ionisation could be one of the most important health breakthroughs in our era.'

To drink or not to drink—That is the question

I often hear people say, 'Don't drink alkaline water, as it prevents digestion.' However, Dr Batmanghelidj and others explain what happens with digestive acids. Acidic stomachs and ulcers are caused by the secreted digestive acid damaging the stomach wall. To prevent this, the stomach wall, which is one cell thick, uses water to form an alkaline buffer layer just above the cells. When we are correctly hydrated, these acids cannot damage our stomach wall.

If we are dehydrated, the stomach lining can be burned by the digestive acids. Stomach pH is about 1.8. To combat this effect, Dr Batmanghelidj recommends drinking two glasses of water thirty minutes before each meal. If this is alkalised water, it is even more effective.

Drinking water with a meal does not create a problem because the water passes straight through into the small intestine (pH 8.2), where it is absorbed into the blood stream and lymphatic system. This ionised water containing negative OH- ions and electrons is then immediately carried around the body to help combat and neutralise disease. Let's also remember that bugs of all kinds thrive in an acidic environment and maintaining correct cell and tissue pH is essential to combating many diseases.

The author of The pH Miracle, Dr Robert Young, says that 'To maintain or restore your body's natural pH balance for optimal health, drink restructured, ionised water which is rich in anti-oxidants and alkaline minerals. Ionised water helps reverse the effects of acid accumulation in the body, the root cause of degenerative diseases and aging.'

Other aspects of our digestive tract also benefit from alkalised water. For example, the job of the gallbladder is to dump adequate amounts of bile into the small intestine to break down the fats in the food that has passed from the stomach. Bile is also intended to change the pH of the food by creating an alkaline tide. However, many people today do not produce enough bile, so fats are often poorly digested and the pH of the small intestine remains too acidic.

The pancreas will only release the enzymes necessary to complete protein digestion if the pH is adequately alkaline, so when bile is inadequate, digestion is severely compromised. Using alkalised water helps rebalance this situation.

Our bodies are super intelligent and any excess of electrons and ions will be neutralised without any side effects.

What to look for in your drinking water

1. ORP (Oxidation Reduction Potential). We want water with a negative ORP which donates free electrons for healing. Water with a –OPR is an antioxidant.

2. Alkalinity. Does it help neutralise the acidity in our bodies from diet, stress and toxins by producing a larger quantity of OH- ions?

3. Is it filtered to eliminate toxic chemicals?

4. Are we getting enough to suit our activity levels? After drinking quality water, it is hard to go back to tap or bottled water. I can taste the chemicals and feel bloated after just a small glass.

A simple summary on water.

Why so much about water?

Well, quite simply, I'm a fan of its amazing benefits and the emerging science behind it all. We take for granted that water is water.

Now you know it's not.

What comes out of your tap is dubious and probably not healing the body. City dwellers especially beware as water that has been recycled many times has to be chemically kept clean. We want to get chemicals out of our bodies, not add more. Look at the many papers on ionised water and enjoy researching as I have. There is substantial research, and Japan is very much leading the way.

Your body wants to find balance and each person is unique in his or her needs. Your own awareness is key to staying healthy and when you start to use ionised water, know that there will be a time of adjustment.

Anyone with a medical condition should check with the manufactures of any device to ensure you are consuming what is ideal for you. For example, those with kidney problems may need to limit the volume they drink. However, Dr Horst Fitzler, a Vascular Surgeon in the US has stated that if you are going to drink water, you should drink the best water! Like many physicians, he endorses the use of ionized water. In the next chapter, we learn about magnetism and how it affects water. This concept of structured or charged water surrounds us and truly needs to be explored as much as possible.

As I said earlier, we live on a beautiful planet where water is the major element. Our bodies are mostly water and it is imperative that we take this theme into account when talking about our self-care. Taking vitamins won't be effective without hydration; detoxifying our cells requires water; energy production is impossible without water! Water is life, healing and natural. Drink the best and care for our rivers and oceans. Nutrition and environmentalism go hand in hand.

What we do to our world we do to ourselves and when we learn to truly nurture our bodies, we will also heal the planet. We are entwined.

CHAPTER 10

Magnetism—
The Earth's Immune System

Over the years, I'd heard of magnetism and tried the odd bracelet without much success and really was a bit sceptical about the wild claims of magnetic mattresses, but nothing could have prepared me for my meeting with Professor Yuri Tkachenko in Dubai. I had no idea about the magnetic technology advancements in medical, environmental or commercial sectors. It left me in awe of one man's dream, dedication and brilliance. His book, Mysteries of Magnetic Energies, is a must-read for anyone interested in this field. It's a modern-day classic, based on hard research and stunning evidence spanning thirty years, with all the findings presented in one book. Professor Yuri, known in the Guinness Book of Records as the Magnet Man, is a graduate of the Leningrad Polytechnic Institute, specialising in power engineering (thermo-dynamics).

He has co-authored more than 500 research works in the field of magnetic technology and as he said to me, 'Once you start looking at magnetic water, you will never look at anything else.' He is clearly an inspired, guided and passionate research scientist on a mission. When I asked him what his dream was, apart from healing people with magnetic technology, he replied, 'To reforest the desert belt in the Gulf region'! Don't laugh—he could do it. He has already succeeded in creating rain in the summer in Dubai, despite the extreme heat.

Professor Yuri's theory is that the magnetic technology creates clouds by injecting negatively-charged oxygen ions (we are back to those powerful electrons again) into the air. As they get higher, their energy and velocity decreases and water molecules in the air attach to them (due to their dipole nature). These molecular complexes (air ions), along with heat energy, rise further and a whole complicated series of events takes place having to do with electrical forces, atmospheric charges, the terrestrial surface and negative charges. Reaching the top troposphere layer, condensation starts and eventually clouds form and rain falls.

As mankind continues to pollute the air and destroy great forests like the Amazon and those in West Africa, we repeatedly enhance the encroachment of desert and drought. The two largest non-polar deserts in the world are the Sahara and Arabian Peninsula. Perhaps Professor Yuri may not see them reforested in his lifetime, but his life's research and dedication to this cause will one day make him a legend—I'm sure of it.

While I was in Dubai meeting amazing people, many parts of England were under water due to some of the worst storms and floods in living memory. I jokingly said to Professor Yuri, 'Can you stop these mega storms?' He quietly replied, 'Yes we can, and we are in discussion with certain governments and meteorological offices at this moment to bring this technology into play to prevent destruction in the future, but as usual, some people are resisting.' Time to wake up again folks; this is not Star Trek or Hollywood, this is hard science and proven technology. Let's use it and help the earth and all her people.

Magnetism is the earth's original force field, shielding the planet from the sun's rays and cosmic forces.

It helps align and realign water—and ours is a planet of water! We need to understand the power of magnetism and what it does. I was privileged to meet the father of magnetic technology, the man behind all the big research teams working with millions of dollars of funding; his technological discoveries change seawater to drinking and irrigation water.

Let's say that again—you can take seawater, magnetise it and use it like fresh water!

Imagine if every lifeboat had a wee funnel and every coastal farm and town could pump sea water through a magnetic pipe to provide drinking water and irrigate super strong and abundant crops or gardens. How many lives would be saved? And while we are on this topic, this technology is also highly effective for converting brackish water to sweet water and eliminating saline soil contamination. Remember, no chemicals are used and no extra power is required.

The power of magnetised water

Professor Yuri says he can adjust the structural properties of water in twenty-one ways, creating water that is biologically alive. This means the water molecules line up in correct sequence, negative to positive, in a sequential pattern and larger clumps of water molecules break down into smaller, individualised H20 molecules. The smaller the water clumps, the easier they are absorbed into the cells. The water's ionic balance is changed. It becomes more fluid, biologically active and has a greater capacity for dissolving substances. This type of water can carry more oxygen and travel through our trillions of cell walls, hydrating, detoxifying and carrying nutrients. This is why it contains such a powerful healing force. We all need to flush out the toxins, hydrate and become oxygenated. As V.I. Vernadsky, founder of the Ukranian Academy of Sciences says, 'Not a single form of life can exist in its own created wastes', but we humans have the ignorance to think that we can!

Professor Yuri explained that each of the different tissues in the body have a different structure of water, e.g. the water inside the blood is different in structure than that the water in the nerve tissues.

> When we drink or cook with chaotic water, the body has to deconstruct it, then recreate structured water to use in all its various processes and cellular structure. This takes energy and time.

When magnetism deconstructs and restructures water into individual ordered molecules, it quickly and easily enters the tissues where it can be used. The trillions of cells throughout the body pull in the water molecules and you will probably find that you don't urinate so quickly after drinking magnetic water.

Normally after drinking lots of tap or bottled water we run to the toilet a lot, which shows us that the water is not being absorbed very well and rather than diluting the blood and lymph the kidneys must excrete it. Your body just can't handle so much unavailable water all at the same time.

Saving the bees

Throughout my travels and during some war zone/trauma healing work, I have seen first-hand the suffering brought on by drought in Africa, India and Australia. So please, anything which alleviates the suffering of life on earth must be brought to the forefront of our awareness.

Over time excessive farming has demineralised the soil and as a result we are now eating fruits and vegetables that have less minerals and vitamins.

Magnetic water helps break down previously unusable clusters of salts and minerals, making them smaller. These microelements can then be absorbed by the plants. Following this principle, basic crops could become super nutritious foods leading to less chronic illness and cellular starvation. In addition, in poor areas of the world, there would simply be more food to eat.

Various international bodies have stated that by 2030 it is suggested that the world will, per capita, be unsustainable regarding its fresh water consumption. Only 2.5 percent of the water on earth is fresh—not saline. Of this, just 1 percent is easily accessible. This leaves approximately 0.007 percent of all water on earth available to nourish its 6.8 billion people. The fresh water is also claimed by industry that uses it, pollutes it and dumps it, and an equal amount goes to households (of which half is used in toilets and sinks, and the same amount is lost through leakage). The remaining largest proportion is used by agriculture for irrigation and livestock, with 40 percent lost en route. This is already a serious global threat to the continuation of the human race.

As one of the greatest understatements ever uttered says: 'Houston, we have a problem.'

A fascinating fact about magnetic water is that bees prefer it. Placing two bowls of water, normal and magnetic, near hives, we can watch as bees and other animals choose magnetic water. We must save the bees, as they practically sustain life as we know it through pollination of our plants, fields and orchards. This chapter is unable to do justice to such a huge topic, but, like all the contents, magnetic water helps lead toward better health.

Professor Yuri described the magnetic field of the earth as its 'immune system'. Destroy it and we also damage the delicate ecosystems, biorhythms and energetic fields that sustain all life.

He has found a way to recreate these magnetic forces, along with fifty-two leading scientific institutes of the Soviet Union and Russia, in such a way as to create healing in humans, animal, plants and the earth.

So far, this kind of technology has been used to treat drinking water and sewage and clean up rivers, sea water, lagoons and lakes. It can also extract the harmful gaseous chlorine out of water and make fish healthier, tastier and bigger. It can change the turbidity of surface water, thus preventing mosquitoes from laying eggs, helping crops to grow bigger, causing plants to need less water and helping water become more biologically active. In daily life, magnetism can also be used to transform the molecules of the water we drink, shower with and with which we irrigate our allotments. Thankfully, there are some simple products available such as the magnetic funnel which I carry around with me to fill my water bottle, kettle or even bath water!

I am choosing to mention just a few examples where magnetism is used outside of the health and wellness field, as I find it quite fascinating to see just who has picked up on this remarkable success story of the twentieth century.

I first heard about magnetism being used in the construction's industry through my friend in Dubai, Jamal Almana. He built his house using magnetic water to mix the cement in order to make it stronger, less corrosive and more stable in extreme conditions.

For over fifteen years, former Soviet Union scientific institutions and organisations have researched the benefits of magnetism in the oil industry, and how it contributes to increased efficiency and cost reduction by improving the operating characteristics of jet fuel.

Magnetism is used to weaken the bonds between paraffin molecules and pipe walls in the oil pipelines. It is also used in the perfume industry to prolong the life and quality of their products. In agriculture, plants and animals are bigger, healthier and less prone to disease and death when magnetic water is used. Farmers who treat their seeds with magnetic water need less for the same yield. It decreases growing times by weeks, reduces disease in the plants by up to 70 percent, increases yield by 40 percent and takes up to 30 percent less water.

Solving environmental pollution

And here's one of my favourite benefits—treating environmental pollution caused by vehicle emissions and industrial pollution. When magnetic systems are installed in vehicles, the toxic fumes and waste are reduced and fuel consumption decreases by 15-25 percent. Incredible, I want one on my car please! If the big boys use it

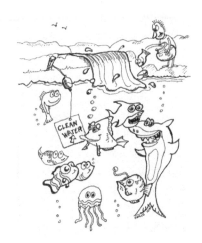

Good water is preferred by all

and it keeps plants, animals, fish and birds healthy, why don't we? Well actually, the short answer to that rhetorical question is, basically, ignorance. Until now we didn't know about it, and now we do. Eureka!

Years ago, the river running through the city of Sochi, Russia and into the Black sea was highly polluted due to heavy industry further upstream. Professor Yuri built a structure that looks like the Thames barrier to magnetise the water. Once the water flowed through it and down into the sea, within twenty-four hours the fish recognised the water had changed and they swam up in such numbers that it was considered a phenomenon. People flocked to the river and saw thousands of fish moving upstream, attracted to the positive water created by the magnets.

By restructuring the water, through magnetism and freeing up H2O molecules from their larger clusters, the fish could benefit from the oxygenation of the water. It's not that there was any more oxygen in the river; it's just that the fish could access it, and given that they need oxygen as much as we do, they quickly swam towards well-oxygenated water. Due to the freeing of H2O molecules from clumps and alignment of the ions, magnetic water does not allow bugs and pathogenic bacteria (anaerobes) to proliferate. The nature of magnetically restructured water with its ordered alignment of positive- to negative-charged molecules further reduces the ability of these pathogens to survive.

In some parts of the world, well water pumped through magnetised pipes provides safe drinking water for the poorest of the poor.

Magnetic water is a naturally occurring gift of life. In far off, distant, inaccessible parts of the world you can find springs that truly have healing water. Most of the water we have today is pretty much dead, through the various mechanical, thermal and chemical 'cleaning' treatments. Holy wells like Lourdes in France and Zamzam near Mecca have renowned healing properties. Sheikh Junaid Khoory was keen to show me a historical book about the Zamzam well and how the stones deep underground are magnetic in nature. As the water flows over them and into the well, it in turn becomes magnetised, leading to much of the purification and healing qualities of the water. Perhaps all healing wells have the same natural magnetic substratum, and along with faith in God, a strong will to heal and some extra minerals and salts like calcium, sulphur and magnesium, our bodies become hydrated, energised and replenished enough to heal.

Treating common conditions

To meet many different challenges, a wide variety of products were created, such as the funnel for magnetising liquids, ear clips or bracelets. When looking to magnetise your water pipes in your home, farm or office, you need an inline device rather than a clamp or barrier magnetic device.

Research from Russia and the United States demonstrates that the following are facilitated by magnetic technology:

- pain relief
- enhanced blood circulation
- healthier hair
- high blood pressure
- joint pain
- swelling and stiffness
- faster healing of wounds and skin conditions
- reduction in gut acidity
- removal of toxins and unwanted salts
- regulation of the menstrual cycle
- clearing of clogged arteries
- healing of burns, cuts, fractures
- improvements in sexual dysfunction
- impotence
- haemorrhoids
- infertility
- coughs
- colds
- headaches
- allergies

If we can balance and heal ourselves with magnetism, or use it as a preventative self-help programme, we are lessening our dependence on pharmaceutical drugs.

In our modern day, unnatural and demagnetised water, molecules have a very different, chaotic pattern, which does not have the same hydration or healing properties as it used to. Professor Yuri explains that everything healthy and balanced in our universe has a sense of order—dark and light, negative and positive, cold and hot. We may have broken the magnetic fields that our forefathers enjoyed, with its bioavailable water that kept all life forms in their optimal states. However, we can now recreate this for ourselves—plants and animals.

The global perspective

I have noticed that the answers to many of our problems today lie in educating each other about all the various available solutions. Each one of us needs to take responsibility and try new things, as Gandhi said, 'My life is an experiment of truth.' What does that mean? Well, to me it means looking at natural solutions that have worked for millions (including those in the past) of people who are staying healthy and beating diseases. Try changing your water, diet and lifestyle.

Frequency and Bioenergy medicine, along with alternative treatments like Ozone which was discovered over 100 years ago, could all have been used instead of antibiotics as the primary anti-bacterial, fungal and viral treatment (with antibiotics being used only when all else fails). It is also the social responsibility of leaders, wealthy individuals and influential people to tackle global issues and to be bold enough to take the necessary steps to implement such powerful scientific advancements on a large scale.

> Imagine what our clinics and hospitals would look like now if natural forms of medicine had been promoted as much as pharmaceutical drugs.

I am an optimist and truly believe that despite all the mistakes, mankind will find ways to bring back the harmony to our planet and our lives. Antibiotics, which were a gift in themselves, could have served humanity for a thousand years if used wisely. Because of their misuse, we face the end of their great era and a desperate need to find alternatives.

Unfortunately, we may have to wait until this health crisis reaches its peak before we realise that together we can create a new, sustainable paradigm for wellness.

CHAPTER 11

Frequency and Bioenergy Technology— Decoded

Living as nature intended is the ideal, yet we have wandered a long way from that. We have the science and technology to recreate those missing or unbalanced elements which would keep us healthy.

> There are devices that will give us photons, electrons and rebalance our energy fields. This is the basis of a new paradigm of health care.

Why do we need technology?

I agree that in a perfect world we wouldn't need technology and devices to help us stay balanced and healthy. However, a perfect world would require the following:

1. No daily chronic stress.

2. A regular diet of mineral rich, organic and free-range foods, with lots of colours, tastes and variety, including intermittent fasting.

3. An emotionally stable, spiritually enriched population that meditates regularly.

4. Going barefoot daily.

5. Spending hours outside in sunlight.

6. Walking as much as possible.

7. Being surrounded by loving families.

8. Eschewing the use of electronic gadgets like phones, laptops and Wi-Fi.

9. Living where there are no radioactive leaks, chemicals dumped in water or landfills, no geopathic stress and so on.

In all honesty, how many of us live like this? Given that we have a less than ideal lifestyle, we can make an effort to live life naturally and allow technology to help us combat the debilitating effects of modern life around us. It's a dichotomy. Technology, like WiFi, is damaging us, but we can also use it to recharge our cells. Laser, Rife, PEMF, Bioresonance, Magnetism and more are there waiting to be used on a daily basis when needed.

Each kind of technology has its own special function and many overlap in both benefit and mechanism. For example, some will work with electromagnetism and micro currents. This makes them difficult to categorise; however, in general, their main function is to increase cell membrane potential (voltage), increase general electron and photon density and, through frequency, boost healthy tissues and denature unwanted microbes. All of which are essential to healing, repair and regeneration.

The leading FAB practitioner in Europe has found that after twenty years of clinical work, not one form of Frequency technology or Bioenergy technique alone will eradicate completely a deep-seated pleomorphic disease like Borrelia. It is the combination of techniques that is successful. For this reason, in Book 2 of this series (coming soon!) I focus on the devices and their practical application throughout the healing journey.

Pulsed electromagnetic field (PEMF)

This technology is very popular with leading national sports teams as it speeds up recovery time. This should not be confused with static magnetic therapy. PEMF therapy has been researched for over thirty years and thousands of papers have been written on its efficacy.

In short, PEMF increases the electrical charge within and around cells and tissues, leading to increased blood supply and, with it, nutrients, oxygen and waste removal.

The electromagnetic pulse goes through the body and shakes the cell walls, providing free electrons while helping cell membrane potential get back to its optimum 80mV cross membrane charge. The pulse also opens cell membrane transport channels. As the channels become unblocked, toxins are released and nutrients rush in.

It is used for conditions such as back pain, fracture healing, arthritis and fibromyalgia. Lying on a PEMF mat increases vitality, which is an aid to healing at home or in a clinical setting. PEMF technology is a valuable asset in Lyme treatment as it helps speed repair of damaged tissues and provides energy to help the exhausted body fight the disease and damage.

Clinics may choose to also have the more expensive and very powerful ringer PEMF devices. These send a shock wave through the tissue, giving medical benefits very rapidly.

Bioresonance

Bioresonance is one of the most effective forms of Technology found in a FAB clinic. It has been used successfully in Germany and other countries for over forty years. This clinical device is employed by thousands of health practitioners, including: medical doctors, dentists and veterinarians. It works to measure the electromagnetic signals coming from the body, filtering out any unhealthy frequencies and sending the healthy signals back. In recent years, China has taken a lead role in the development and use of these devices in government-run hospitals.

Working off the premise that cells communicate using photon radiation their resonant frequencies can be enhanced with frequency-based devices. If the Bioresonance device finds you have discordant or unhealthy frequencies stemming from microbes or sick cells, it will invert them, play them back to the body and neutralise the stressful frequencies. It works a bit like noise-cancelling headphones for use on aeroplanes. These devices are especially useful for detecting and dealing with all kinds of microbes, allergens, toxins, chemicals, heavy metals, e-smog and food sensitivities.

People who have Borrelia and co-infections respond well to Bioresonance treatments and your local therapist should have the vials which carry the frequencies of all the microbes and toxins you wish to neutralise and eliminate. Bioresonance can also be used to strengthen various parts of the body and re-educate immune cells to find invading microbes.

It is a very good natural form of healing, not just for reducing the stress or toxic load in chronic diseases, but also for tackling day to day conditions such as colds and flu, hay fever, digestive disorders and back pain.

Rife machines and zappers

Knowing that all things have their own frequencies, from bugs to liver cells, we can use specific frequencies to boost tissues and kill or denature unwanted organisms and cells. This is the main concept behind the research and work of Dr Royal Rife,

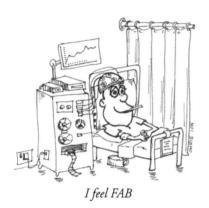

I feel FAB

Hulda Clark and Alan Baklayan, along with many others. Over the past eighty years, the specific frequencies that denature micro-organisms from Candida to Bartonella have been identified and programmed into devices. They are delivered to the body via a number of ways from neon tubes to coils. Most of these devices are expensive and the more powerful ones are used in clinics. For those who can afford them, they are also a valuable tool for home use.

They can cause large scale microbial die off and, with it, strong Herx reactions as the body tries to handle a sudden surge of dead microbes.

> Microbes ingest heavy metals and chemical toxins, which are released into the body fluids as the organism dies. This is one of the reasons the correct approach is needed when using Rife technology.

You simply can't just blast the body and expect to heal—many chronically ill people make this mistake and wonder why they are not recovering. Other frequencies which strengthen the organs are used before and after killing bacteria and viruses.

There are many types of Rife machines on the market, from cheapies made in China to larger, more powerful ones individually produced to order. Budget, experience and usage all impact what kind you would need to choose should you be unwell with Lyme or similar diseases.

Zappers

Simple ones are very cheap and deliver a couple of electromagnetic frequencies for general use. Good for wearing on the go in the car, train or plane as a protective booster for the immune system or simply around the house.

The more advanced zappers are designed to deliver a range of frequencies and act like a mini Rife machine and Bioresonance device. Some can also deliver micro-currents for pain relief. They are considered supplementary to clinical treatments and effective for home use and are ideal for people with limited finances and for those who cannot get to a Bioresonance practitioner, require back up treatments at home between clinical care or those without a larger Rife machine. I have a German one and carry it everywhere and most of my family and friends want to use it too!

Light—Practical applications

Clinics use Laser therapy (photobiomodulation) and Biophoton therapy to treat the lack of photon energy and disturbed photon communication. In Borellia-focussed FAB clinics, light is used to draw microbes out of cells (where they hide) and into the interstitial spaces to be attacked by a patient's own immune cells.

Laser devices direct light into joints, muscles and organs, aiming to improve vitality through increased electron and photon activity, leading to greater cellular metabolism and healing. They work in the visible red light range from about 650 to 780 nanometers and the invisible infrared spectrum of over 780 nm. This kind of treatment can be used in both acute injuries (many sports or physio clinics have them) and for chronic conditions.

Light treatments also benefit those with Lyme disease with laser treatments being used to open cysts and biofilms and bring light and healing information to affected areas. Spirochete's can travel deep into organs and tissues, such as the nerves, brain, joints and bones.

Meanwhile, in mainstream research, photomedicine is leaping forward with a possible new direction by using green laser light for photochemical tissue bonding. Whichever way we look at it, using light to heal is here to stay.

Infrared saunas can be a valuable tool in Lyme disease with some companies offering small half saunas for home use. Lasers can be used to stimulate acupuncture points and stimulate the meridians. Infrared treatments are also given for the alleviation of pain, inflammation, immunomodulation and wound healing.

Biophoton therapy devices are used to measure and assess levels of light in the cells and how discordant or harmonious it is. Good ones also have the ability to locate a block in the energy flow or tissue where there is less light.

Devices work to gather information on discordant frequencies and bring it back through the machine via a biofeedback system. The devices correct and send them back into the body. More advanced Biophoton devices can be programmed with homoeopathic nosodes which carry the inverted frequency to the hidden microbe, neutralising the bacteria.

Information field technology

Another emerging field in recent years has been the development of computer-based technology that uses special programmes to scan and measure areas of imbalance throughout the body. Along with the pure physical aspect, these devices record emotional, mental and spiritual vibrations—often with remarkable accuracy. They are tapping into the holographic information field of the person and then, by using the biofeedback principle, sending a message of healing and wholeness back to these layers. This information field technology seeks to record information taken from the quantum level. By measuring or 'seeing' what's happening in our holographic quantum field, these devices interpret wellness or disharmony at many levels, from molecules to chakras and so on.

The more advanced devices can detect tens of thousands of frequencies that may be influencing health, from parasites to minerals, chakras to emotions. Many of the better FAB clinics have one or two Information Field devices and some companies produce a home-use version. They come into their own with Lyme disease when they are used to find the specific frequencies of disease microbes, which are then transferred to a Rife machine to be neutralised.

This is an ever-changing and often bewildering field of health care. For more information on specific devices mentioned in the book and used in the specialised Lyme FAB clinic in Europe, please visit www.pauletteagnew.com.

CHAPTER 12

Staying Healthy—
It's easy when you know how

Finding solutions to our daily problems lies in learning and application, along with a good dose of trial and error! We are all in a constant process of change, growth and decay, so stay open to trying new things, especially when it comes to staying young and healthy. Don't forget to think about what you think! Your emotions and thoughts (including memories) are pulsing messages to your body and the greater whole of creation. Healthy, happy thoughts nourish the physical structure.

Here is my ideal action plan to harmonise our light bodies through Frequency and Bioenergy.

Air

- Get an air ioniser for your office or indoor work spaces. Should you live in an air-conditioned apartment, use one there too.
- Open windows and doors as often as possible throughout the day to bring in fresh air and health-giving, negative ions to your home or work. Sleep with a window open.
- Learn pranayama or deep breathing exercises to increase oxygen content of the cells to beat infections and create optimum vitality.
- Walk or cycle to work where possible. Find sports and hobbies that take you outside and breathe deeply, appreciating the air and winds around you.

Everyone needs a different approach, diet or exercise regime to suit their constitution but the basics are essential, such as good water, electrons and photons.

Earth

- Go out into nature with bare feet (or whole body) and connect to the earth and water (walk, sit or lie on the grass/earth). Wild places like beaches, forests and mountains are highly charged. If you live in a city, go find a garden or park and fill up on electrons, ideally on a daily basis.
- Try an activity like Tai Chi or Yoga to keep the body supple and stimulate the meridians or energy channels. When it comes to our mechanical body parts, if you don't use them, you lose them!

Water

- Use a high-quality water ioniser
- Drink only filtered water and, if possible, filter it before showering and bathing.
- Eat foods with high water content like fresh fruits and vegetables, avoiding prepacked meals, dried foods and sweet soda type drinks.
- Older people can often lose their thirst receptors and tend to drink less water as a result. Ensure you take in enough water for your age and environmental conditions.
- Flying is very dehydrating. Keep the water up and alcohol down on aeroplanes.
- Coffee and tea are not water and some herbal teas are also diuretic.
- Use oils on your skin to moisturise and ensure your diet contains enough fresh oils in the correct combination.

Light and photons

- Eat only biological/organic foods where possible. Ensure they're fresh, slow-cooked (some raw) and not genetically modified.
- Ensure your diet contains sun-filled fruit, seeds, nuts and vegetables.
- See the next section of the book to learn about ideal dietary requirements, especially oils.

- Go out into natural light (sunshine) every day. Try to have some time in the light without sun block and allow your skin to absorb photons.

Earth magnetism

- Use Frequency devices in clinics and at home to strengthen yourself and your immune system to effectively beat disease and infections.
- If you are a city dweller, take weekends and holidays in nature.
- Cars, trains, planes and steel buildings are like faraday cages—insulating you. As often as you can, go outside and put your bare hands and feet on the earth.
- Protect yourself from dangerous e-smog with protectors on your smart phones, tablets and computers, along with car and house protection.
- Use magnetic mats or PEMF devices at home to maintain cellular vitality and efficiency (as discussed in the next section).

My sincere wish is that by reading and exploring ideas presented in this book you will embark on a journey of discovering the nature of life and see a beautiful interconnection between yourself and the world you live in.

In Part 2 of this book you will find out how the 100 trillion cells in your body coexist and sustain your life. You will learn how to bring and maintain balance within your body by keeping individual cells clean and nourished.

PART 2

Bioenergy
Detox, Repair and Renew

From the invisible world of particles and waves, let's step into the visible structure of our cells, bodies and biochemistry.

When cells become overloaded and toxic, illness begins.

CHAPTER 13

100 Trillion Cells

By now you have a good understanding of your invisible, holographic, energy body and the need to nourish and protect the essence of who you truly are.

Although in principle going out barefoot into the garden in the sunlight should make you super healthy and balanced, it's not the be-all and end-all solution. One has to consider numerous other factors to reach full health.

It doesn't matter how much light or energy we bathe ourselves in, if the body is toxic and lacks essential nutrients, we cannot repair or renew effectively. Microorganisms, parasites and bacteria just love a dirty, low oxygenated, acidic cellular environment. In fact, they thrive in it!

We are a community of 100 Trillion cells.

Why focus on cells? Because we are the sum of all of our cells! To prevent the bad guys taking over and to be super charged humans, we need every cell to be working at its best. We need to eliminate the factors that make our bodies a juicy home for the nasty microbes to breed. When I look back in time, I can see, with all honesty, how my pre-Lyme lifestyle and dietary habits were abysmal. I can see now that my poor cells had malnutrition and were swamped in waste from bad dietary choices. They also had to endure a deep, unresolvable emotional crisis combined with constant long-haul flying, which caused more stress and dehydration.

In short, I had created a vibrational nightmare for them, and when they complained, I just didn't listen to the warning signs. Soon various bad bugs were breeding and spreading. Help was sorely needed. The time had come to implement a rescue mission.

You are the captain of your intergalactic space station

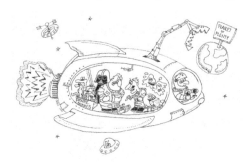

Space, the final frontier

A vast hidden world lies within, consisting of trillions of cells and microbes of many different kinds.

If we had super-power vision and could look inside each other, we would see this teeming mass of microbes and human cells, all co-existing (mostly symbiotically) like an intergalactic, deep space station. I loved watching the popular sci-fi TV series 'Babylon 5' and imagining my body as a spaceship, a vessel which hosts all kinds of weird and wonderful inhabitants! This spaceship analogy can help us visualise this concept and appreciate what exactly we are doing to ourselves.

We can imagine how the different departments inside ourselves host unique 'dwellers', each quite distinctive in appearance, purpose and ability. All these organisms are protected by our sealed outer casing, our skin or hull. The ship needs to maintain a regular intake of nutrients and oxygen as well as ensuring that the waste or rubbish is expelled from the ship.

To continue to thrive, repair and reproduce, our hard-working crew (the cells and microbes) also needs minerals, good oils, light and cleanliness. Collectively, the crew is designed to keep the spaceship operational from birth to death.

They will only cause problems and threaten the ability of the spaceship to operate if ignored, abused or given poor quality provisions and working conditions.

Remember, you are the captain of your ship and you determine the conditions your workers must endure.

Some of the most common moment-by-moment bad policy decisions made on the bridge and sent down to the crew are those concerning nutrition. Without awareness and care, it's all too easy to feed our worker cells hazardous amounts of sugar (or high carbohydrate foods), as well as those containing bad fats. Meanwhile our cells are also suffering from lack of good quality water (and remembering that herbal teas are not water), acid-forming foods, toxic chemicals from all sources, lowered oxygen intake through poor posture, insufficient breath awareness and lack of fresh air. Pretty poor working conditions, wouldn't you say?

What goes in must come out

Most people like a clean and tidy home and at least throw out their rubbish! This principle of good housekeeping also applies to the inside of our body where our hard-working cells also require the same. When I've had the privilege of traveling to parts of rural India and Africa, meeting local people in their mud huts, what struck me the most was their attention to cleanliness. They may squat to cook over a fire and sleep on cow dung floors, but they scour their cooking pots, boil their water, beat their clothes ruthlessly in the river and forever sweep their floors. I've never seen food remains left lying around to fester in corners and doors are always left open to allow in sunlight and fresh air.

The challenge facing more advanced nations is the obsession with the 'outside world'. In striving for materialistic success, wealth and comfort, we have forgotten the most important part of ourselves: that which lies within.

I think this is because the world outside our spaceship becomes too captivating or demanding and we, the captains, don't think it's important enough to dedicate the time, money or energy needed for those crucial inner jobs like throwing out the waste (detoxification).

Let's face it, dealing with the rubbish bin, blocked waste disposal units or sewage pipes is an icky job that most people avoid at all costs. However, toxic waste will eventually build up and that eventually poisons the whole ship. Detrimental and aggressive microbes will thrive, breed and accumulate in large numbers, eventually taking over the dirtier parts of the ship. If that happens, it means the captain was not taking care of his immunity, causing his security forces to become too weak to control or dispose of the bad guys.

You are always in charge

The captain can become so engrossed in his or her 'mission' that they may fail to notice the many small changes in quality of the supplies (nutrition) being brought in. Full and fast lifestyles can stop you from noticing the many seemingly unconnected complaints of your workers and departments. Buying cheap, processed foods with the intention of saving money or time only costs more

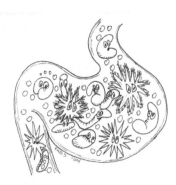

Microbes thrive in a dirty home

in the long run, and pharmacies are full of drugs to soothe the associated symptoms and complaints of your worker inhabitants—without solving the real problem.

Perhaps it's time to use our more luxurious, choice-filled lives to assist in caring for ourselves and not destroying (without thinking) this precious body. Unlike a car or spaceship, we can't just trade the old, bashed one in and get a new one halfway through our life. In the end, no one can survive long-term on poor care and resources and the workers will eventually rebel or go on strike! How else will they get the attention of their leader?

Further complications arise over time, because as each new generation of cells is manufactured using lower-grade materials, they inevitably get weaker.

Finally, we end up with a body (our spaceship), that has a weak immune system, low energy output, poor communication pathways and a dysfunctional sewage system—and we wonder why!

Some captains care deeply for their ship and crew; others don't and theirs become battered and bruised by choice. These captains end up frequenting the many intergalactic substations for regular repairs, which are costly, often brutal and sometimes require the loss of parts of their ship. To be honest, it took the extreme Lyme disease and an almost complete shutdown of my ship to wake me up and force me to listen to my cellular inhabitants. I hope you don't have to reach rock bottom before taking charge and befriending yours.

Outside the content of this book, but equally important, are our thoughts, emotions and spiritual beliefs. They can be considered the software or master computer programme, which ultimately controls what happens at physical and energy levels. If we have programmed our bodies to act and react in certain ways over many years or even decades, a change of mind one day will not automatically create spontaneous healing.

It will take time, patience, repetitive actions, feelings and thoughts to reprogram the whole system. But just imagine how fabulous the new you will be!

Becoming aware and supporting the needs of the trillions of tiny individual cells and microbes, which collectively make up our inner symbiotic community, will make us strong, happy, vibrant and truly alive.

With a fully functioning space station, we will face every opportunity, challenge or change with power and clarity, no matter how far we travel.

Wellness is determined by a number of factors. In addition to the light, voltage, water and oxygen we have already discussed, we also need the correct nutrients, strong mini-generators (mitochondria) and healthy cell membranes. As we have just seen with the spaceship analogy, a good waste removal and drainage system is essential for detoxification.

Gut bugs—the master controllers

Microbes living in and on us are partly responsible for our overall health and aid basic essential bodily tasks, such as breaking down food. If their number or proportion gets out of balance, it can lead to many conditions, such as depression and autoimmune diseases.

Some microbes are considered pathogenic but do not always cause disease. In fact, many have some beneficial effects. It is the condition of the intra- and extracellular terrain, and the state of the gut in particular, that appears to trigger imbalances and allows microbes to flourish.

The human gastrointestinal tract is colonised by approximately 1011 symbiotic, commensal and pathogenic microbes (bacteria, virus and fungi) per gram of intestinal content. Studies show we are in fact 90 percent nonhuman DNA! Studying this collective population called a 'microbiome' or 'microbiota' is one of the fastest growing fields in medicine. The Human Microbiome Project launched in 2007 by the National Institutes of Health is very much leading the way.

Lita Proctor, coordinator of this programme, says, 'We need to know what is their role (these microorganisms), what are they doing for us and how can we support that role if it helps our health.'

Dr. Jeffry Katz, medical director of the inflammatory bowel disease centre at University Hospitals Cleveland Medical Centre in Ohio says, 'There are lines of evidence, some from animal models but also some human evidence that the gut bacteria are going to be very important for a number of human health conditions. It's really a field at its infancy.'

Although it is considered an emerging field of scientific study, some of the oldest forms of medicine, such as Ayurveda, focus on the gut as the beginning of healing and are imperative to good healthcare.

> What the evidence indicates is that in order to heal ourselves and stay in top form, we need to keep our gut correctly inhabited.

And when we have a healthy digestive tract, the good gut microbes not only produce enzymes that help digest food, but they also produce certain essential vitamins. In humans, it has been shown that members of the gut microbiota are able to synthesise vitamin K as well as most of the water-soluble B vitamins, such as: biotin, cobalamin, folates, nicotinic acid, pantothenic acid, pyridoxine (Vitamin B6), riboflavin and thiamine.

Our digestive tract, from mouth to anus, appears to be the master controller of the whole-body microbiome. When communities of microbes are kept in balance and in the right proportions, we remain well. If we upset that balance with poor diet, stress, toxins etc., the balance is lost, aggressive microbes get out of hand and we become ill. Many studies show the active role of intestinal microbiota in the immune system with probiotics used

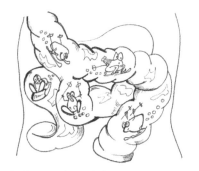

Which part of you did you say is human?

in the treatment of various immune diseases. Dan Peterson, assistant professor of pathology at the Johns Hopkins University School of Medicine says, "A huge proportion of your immune system is actually in your GI tract."

During a natural birth, some microbes from the mother's birth canal will enter the baby's mouth and become part of the baby's immune system development during the first two years. To aid the development of C-section babies' immunity, a process called 'seeding' is gaining popularity, whereby a saline-soaked swab of the mother's vagina just before birth is gently rubbed on the baby's skin, eyes and inside its mouth. Other pioneering work with cancer patients in some research hospitals involves storing samples of their microbiomes for reintroduction after chemotherapy in order to help rebuild immunity.

Antony Hynes, in an action-packed video interview with me at the Royal Society of Medicine, described the interrelationship between the gut, diet and cellular membrane health. He explained that it is possible to heal a damaged blood brain barrier, brain fog, cognitive problems, memory loss and even Gulf War Syndrome through nutrition. One of the points he made in our discussion about mental health was that 90 percent of serotonin is made in the gut. He also went on to explain how the friendly gut bacteria strains also produce dopamine, gabba and noradrenaline.

In a nutshell, our gut biome is hugely important for reducing the burden of inflammatory molecules and improving neurotransmitter receptor function, as well as helping detoxification.

If you are experiencing challenges with mood swings, depression and emotional dips, it's time to look at your diet. I know it's hard to think about making a healthy meal with chronic fatigue and being super sick, but, in fact, it makes a massive difference in all areas of our recovery. Try to eat about twenty different kinds of foods each day to broaden the range of your microbiome. I love to help mine by picking and eating super foods found growing in the hedgerows on the side of quiet, country roads.

CHAPTER 14

Happy Cell Essentials

There are many groups of cells in our bodies constituting different tissues, organs and systems. Each set has a different job to do but they all have the same things in common. They need to create energy, undergo repairs and make new cells.

To keep all the of the cells healthy we require a number of key electrolytes and trace minerals, including: Sodium, Calcium, Potassium, Magnesium and Sulphur. Water and Oxygen are the other dominant ingredients. Also essential are Iron, Manganese, Selenium, Copper, Chromium, Iodine, Chloride, Boron and Molybdenum.

Barbara Wren, founder of the College of Natural Nutrition in the UK, explains that, predominantly in the daytime, electrolytes sodium and calcium move into the cells and to keep a balance, potassium and magnesium move out. At night, this is reversed. When sodium and calcium build up in our cells, we start to feel tired and the body gets the message to lie down and rest or sleep. During this time, they return to the outside of the cells and potassium and magnesium travel back into the cells. Water molecules also flow into the cells along with oxygen, whilst waste and carbon dioxide flow out.

Inside every cell we have little energy factories called mitochondria. Within each of these mitochondria a series of complex mechanisms occurs, which create energy for life. The Krebs cycle is probably the best known biochemical pathway where Adenosine Triphosphate (ATP) is created. This is the storehouse of power, our own mini suns or super batteries. In order to produce energy, ATP breaks down into Adenosine Diphosphate (ADP), releasing electrons which, as we have seen, are essential to the electricity of the body. Low electrons, low voltage, low energy.

Like your electric toothbrush at home, the battery runs slow when it is running out of charge. To get more power, we simply plug the toothbrush back into the main supply where it stores energy until the next teeth cleaning experience. Our bodies are just the same.

> When we fill up with electrons and highly charged ATP molecules, we are ready to run that marathon!

To produce ATP, glucose molecules enter the cell and are broken down in a process called glycolysis. Making two pyruvate molecules, which then creates two ATP and 2 NADH +H$^+$, but this is nowhere near enough for healthy bodies. If oxygen is not around, pyruvate can be turned into lactic acid. All athletes know that feeling of hitting the wall. Or have you ever had to make a mad dash to catch a train, run out of breath and gotten cramps?

If we do not oxygenate the body through correct breathing and regular daily exercise, the pyruvate can be used by all those bugs, yeasts, moulds and other anaerobes to make ethanol and CO2, which in turn makes the cell acidic. Naturally, we don't want this. Ethanol is also a solvent and damages the cell membrane; it breaks down the phospholipid bilayer and denatures the protein by breaking the hydrogen bonds.

Assuming we breathe well, exercise daily and have a healthy transport system (the blood), all of our cells will have oxygen, which travels along with pyruvate into the mitochondria to enter the Krebs citric acid cycle and make large amounts of energy in the form of ATP. To complete the detoxification journey, the waste products need to be taken out of the cells into the extracellular fluids: blood and lymph. From there they are taken to the liver and kidneys for removal.

The drainage system

The lymphatic fluid bathes all the tissues, maintaining fluid balance. It carries infection-fighting white blood cells throughout the body to be filtered in the lymph nodes and lymphatic organs (spleen and thymus). It is also responsible for absorbing and transporting fatty acids and fats from the digestive system. Truly one of the most crucial systems to maintaining health and vitality.

The reason I elaborate on this topic is to emphasise in particular the importance of correct breathing. Low oxygenation of tissues limits the production of ATP and hence limits energy.

Low Oxygen = Low Energy

My "Beyond Fatigue" home programme is especially designed for oxygenating the cells using breathing and movement exercises. It is ideal for people with Lyme and Chronic Fatigue.

The Lymphatic system is an essential part of detoxifying the body. Lymphatic fluid does not get pumped around the body by the heart. It needs the contraction of muscles and the movement of the diaphragm to get it flowing. No exercise, no drainage. Massage helps of course, but who can afford to get hours of treatment on the couch each day? Our natural daily movements—walking, bending, squatting, twisting, arm swinging and deep breathing—are all designed to detox the body. Taking time to exercise is essential to wellness. Sitting all day in a car, office chair or sofa will alone make you sick. Move and you will live longer.

I've been teaching therapeutic movement and breath work for twenty-five years around the world and I am fully convinced it aids healing. A well-designed movement programme will help you squeeze, flex and stimulate every part of your body, shifting the lymph and toxins in the tissues and stimulating fresh blood flow to the organs. And before you say, 'But I'm so tired and sick I can't move', there is a lot you can do lying down, sitting or standing in one spot! I know what it's like to lie on a sofa all day, barely able to walk to the toilet and, yes, even then you can do a huge amount to help yourself get well.

If you are reading this book for general interest, use movement as a preventative.

If you have a disease, then you must move. I know it's hard, but without moving you will stagnate more and more.

If you are really incapacitated, ask a friend, family member or therapist to move your body and limbs for you. If you have any strength in you, start to do a few restorative movements every day. Correct, gentle movement always increases energy, Prana and Chi (light and electrons) around the body and organs. Focusing the mind and breath along with some specific actions is hugely regenerative.

Hydrate and flush out the toxins

Detoxification is a key aspect in all natural healing protocols.

We can help ourselves by making sure we are properly hydrated, which is crucial to flushing out waste from the cells. Water is the basis of all cellular function and the hydrogen H+ and Hydroxyl OH- components are used in almost every molecular compound and transformation in the body. Water is used in the breakdown of sugars and fats. It is the basis of the acid/alkali balance in all cellular fluids; molecules arrange themselves in the body as either water-loving or water-repelling. When we have a lot of waste in the cells, blood or lymph, we need water to help alkalise and create fluidity. If we are not correctly hydrated, we will not effectively detox.

The liver does most of the detoxification, creating bile, which is emptied into the duodenum and out of the body though the faeces. Some waste comes out in our urine, some as phlegm or mucous and quite a lot via the skin as sweat. We also detox through the breath during respiration. Do you notice if it smells when you sweat? Do you prevent sweaty armpits with antiperspirants? If so, stop now. Use only a natural deodorant if you must and preferably don't use anything, if possible. If you smell, your body is throwing out waste and it's a wake-up call, but don't stop this elimination.

If you are at home, then simply wash under your arms a few times a day and, if need be, change your shirt. Should you have the luxury of the sea nearby, jump in for a swim each day. Even better if you live in a warm climate, as we sweat and detox through the pores more in the heat! The salty sea water helps draw out toxins from the skin, which is one of the reasons we feel better after a beach holiday (assuming it's not a crazy boozy one!). If you cannot jump into the sea, consider a warm Epsom salts bath once a week.

Count your poos—Better out than in!

The second main way of clearing the sewage out of the body is one's poo. Yes, that is really an important subject. Call it what you will, you need to go every day. Ayurveda says you should eliminate on waking or around breakfast time and after each main meal. If you eat three big meals a day, that's ideally three big trips to the toilet. Many naturopaths and functional medicine practitioners will encourage the use of enemas to help eliminate waste as part of your treatments. Don't be shocked, you get used to them!

Stools should be neither dry and hard nor runny and have a general brownish colour and come out easily, no straining, etc.

If you are not going regularly, where is all that waste being kept?

Well it builds up in the acres of folded digestive tract, mostly in the large intestine. It can be there for years and becomes almost black. If you haven't had a full colonic (a thorough cleansing of the colon in a colonic treatment centre), try one. Although if you have a chronic condition, check with your naturopath or lead therapist first as it may just be too much for your body right now. If you are constipated at all, it's a sure sign you may well be dehydrated.

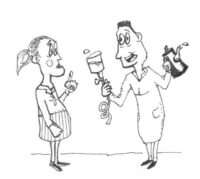

Coffee, or clear out Madam?

The body draws excess moisture out of the faeces in the large intestine to help hydrate the body. If you are not taking in enough high-quality water, it will lead to dry stools. On this topic, one more point to think about, if you have years of old sewage backed up in your body, don't you think the toxins will seep through back into the body through the gut lining? The answer is yes, it does, adding more strain to the body. If you are not 'going' (to the toilet), the toxins are still going somewhere!

Detox thoughts and feelings

Apart from the physical aspects of detoxification, we also need to reflect upon and respect the need for emotional, psychological and spiritual detoxification. Anyone who has been through a healing crisis will tell you they went through 'dark' or difficult emotional releases. Our thoughts, feelings and beliefs are totally related to our wellness. You will find a lot of material around today to help you look at pain, stress or trauma, which imprints on our cells as dis 'ease'. The word itself says we are in a state of dis-ease within ourselves.

When we carry unhappy or agitated vibrations in the form of feelings, emotions and thoughts, we are affecting cellular vibration.

Body-mind-emotional healing is holistic. Old traditions through today's modern health regimes have guidelines to aid us so that we can see our loss of inner harmony. The Chinese system is aware of this and discusses how different parts of the body reflect different mind-sets. Grief, for example, is mirrored in the lungs, and fear in the kidneys. Toxic emotions lead to toxic cells and tissues, leading to troubles in the liver. It may take many years to manifest, as the body is remarkably resilient and tries desperately to heal against all odds, but eventually deeply harboured pain and traumatic memories will manifest.

All life is vibration and our trillions of cells and microbes thrive in a loved, happy, appreciated, clean and well-nourished body.

CHAPTER 15

The Intelligent Protective Barrier

Cell membranes consist of a phospholipid bilayer, which is primarily made of fat. This construction allows the transport of nutrients into the cell and waste out. It also creates a protective layer, which prevents water loss and consequently dehydration of the cell. The cell membranes mostly use longer chain fats taken from our diet. A fat molecule looks like a head with two legs or tails.

The fats in the cell membrane are a crucial player in the electrical currents and energy of the body in a number of ways. The middle of the layer (hydrophobic) acts as storage (like a battery) for ions, whilst the positively-charged heads sticking out into the extracellular space attract and gather electron clouds around them. This is why the surface of cells appears negatively charged.

In recent years fat has been given bad press and we were sold the concept that eating fat will make us overweight and give us heart disease. This is incorrect. It's eating the wrong fats (many fats in processed food have effectively become plastic) causes the cells to starve.

The cells then shout at us to eat more to get energy, so we reach for sugar and fast carbs. We can't use these 'plastic' fats as fuel, for construction of the cells or to do all their other important jobs. On top of this, the body must break them down to make them safely eliminate, which takes even more energy. After a while, the liver and pancreas just can't keep up with processing these abnormal compounds and send them into safe storage. This adds to the 'fat' layers around our organs and under the skin.

Although, finally the tables are turning and the importance of good, old-fashioned fat or oil is coming back into favour. Enough articles are being written and research confirmed by natural health specialists for the population to realise fats are not the evil component lurking in our diets.

Fresh raw oil is the king of nutrition.

It carries huge chains of free electrons, all of which help charge and heal the body.

The phospholipid molecule consists of a polar head containing a phosphate group and a fatty acid tail composed of a string of carbons and hydrogens. It has a kink in one of the chains because of its double-bond structure.

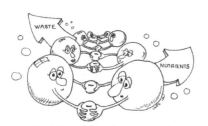

Healthy cell membranes are the secret key to vitality

The phospholipids naturally organize themselves in a double bilayer. It is a highly impermeable structure; therefore, pathways must be built into the membrane that control the flow of molecules in and out. When the cell is hungry, it signals for more nutrients to be sent in, and when it has waste, that gets pushed out. Fats are fluid, which allows the cell membrane to be dynamic. Bruce Lipton in his book *Biology of Belief* calls them liquid crystal, which is a really good way to visualise them. In another great book, *Healing is Voltage* by Dr. Jerry Tennant, there's a further explanation of how the phospholipid bilayer is both a microprocessor and a transistor.

Electrons, molecules and charged ions such as potassium and calcium are constantly flowing in and out of each cell. Healthy phospholipid membranes have the ability to store electrons for rainy days and some of those liquid crystal phospholipids are also responsible for transporting photons into the cells; that's awesome!

When you get chronically ill, it often stems from the cell membranes being undernourished.

Cell membranes can lose their electron storage ability after years of eating margarine, fried foods and processed food like cakes and biscuits.

The phospholipid bilayer by then will be partially made of inert trans fats.

Cell membrane transport systems

To facilitate the flow of molecules through this watertight, sealed membrane, each cell also creates channel or tubes made of proteins (built from amino acids) called Integral Membrane Proteins (IMPs). The middle section of the protein's amino acids is hydrophobic (water fearing) and the ends that stick in and out of the cell are hydrophilic (water loving). They exist as receptor proteins and effector proteins.

Receptors are like antennae and are constantly getting messages from the inside or outside of the cell. They recognise and communicate via the physical reality of molecules and they can pick up vibrational signals, light, sound and radio. Given the context of this book, this is a very important point to remember. When a particular molecule comes along, the protein chain changes structure and the message is delivered to the other end. Each cell membrane has thousands of these IMPs on the lookout for a huge variety of messages which are sending signals in and out of the cells.

The other type of protein, the 'effectors', channel molecules into the cell and waste out. Let's look at the day-night cycle I mentioned earlier, where sodium and potassium are exchanged through the cell walls in one particular protein passageway. Three positively-charged sodium ions are pumped out of the cell and, at the same time, two positively-charged potassium molecules are delivered into the cell. The outer side of the cell wall becomes slightly more positive for a moment again, creating another way of attracting electrons to the cells to power them up. The cell nucleus is kept positively-charged, hence creating a battery effect, a self-replicating power source. We really are a living dynamo when we keep the conditions right.

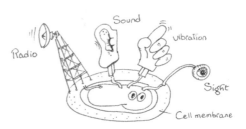

You have your own Internet, smart phones and WiFi!

These effector proteins have other functions, such as helping with the shape of the cells. Some are enzymes, which catalyse the breakdown or manufacture of necessary molecules. They use energy from ATP to do this. These movements of molecules in and out of the cell, in and out of the mitochondria and nucleus, all need energy. This is just to keep us alive, and we haven't run a marathon yet!

All in all, there is a lot going on. The cell is recognising its environment and doing something about it, second by second. This is an intelligent process and our trillions of cells are like mini brains. Block these protein doorways in and out and the cell dies. Change our dietary fats and the membrane can hardly function; dehydrate it and acids build up. Lose contact with nature's ions and there is no power. No wonder those little Lyme spirochetes, other microbes and parasites can find their way into our unhappy cells and start to take over.

American biologist Bruce Lipton concluded that "the cells' operations are primarily moulded by its interaction with its environment, not by its genetic code.' That's powerful stuff because what he's saying is that every single cell in our body is changing according to what we eat, drink, breathe, say, do, think, feel and believe about ourselves. Our bodies are the sum of what we build them with on a daily basis.

Each cell is replaced every few days, weeks, or at the most, months. You are not the person you were a year ago—quite literally. All your cells are new. Do you want to be a new person? Do you want to rebuild the space station and make it a great place to live? If the answer is yes, then we know how. We should fill it with light, air, ions, exercise, water, minerals and fresh nutrients.

The Golden Seven:
Light, air, ions, exercise, water, minerals and fresh nutrients.

These 'Golden Seven' are nature's gifts, enabling humanity to exist indefinitely. And for those of you with a garden, allotment, green house or space for a few pots, you could be growing some of your own organic food too.

I love the phrase, 'If you keep doing the same things over and over, you will get the same results.' And the other one: 'What's the definition of madness? To do the same thing every day and expect a different result.'

CHAPTER 16

Cell Repair and Renewal

All of our 100 Trillion cells need a lot of fat to make healthy cell membranes. We need a mixture of essential fatty acids (EFAs) in our diet, as the body cannot manufacture them. Fatty acids constitute about 25 percent of our body weight and the brain is mostly made of fats, as are the nervous system and liver.

There are three types of omega 3 oils: Alpha-linolenic acid (ALA), found in flax oil, chia seeds, sea buckthorn, walnut and hemp oil, and Eicosapentaenoic acid (EPA) and Docosahexaenoic acid (DHA), commonly found in fish oils, egg oil, squid oils and krill oil.

Omega 6 oils include: Linoleic acid (LA), which is found in nut and seed oils, e.g. hempseed as well as in spirulina, wheat germ and legumes, Gamma–linolenic acid (GLA), which is found in black currant and evening primrose oil, and Dihomo-gamma-Linolenic Acid (DGLA) found in mother's milk. In turn, these get converted to arachidonic acid (AA) and prostaglandins, which are vital as they feed into the endocrine/hormonal system and serotonin production.

Omega 9 (oleic acid) can be produced by the body so it is not classified as an essential fatty acid. It is mostly found in olive oil, avocados and nut oils.

The brain demands omega 3 and 6 oils, which have high numbers of double-carbon bonds, which in turn attract electron clouds, in effect ensuring the brain

99

has a plentiful supply of voltage and energy. Our bodies are incredibly clever and, when given the right conditions, really want to be well. The darker, colder and more northern your abode, chances are you will need more omega 3 to compensate for the lack of light, as the electron clouds in oils also attract photons. People living in very hot countries, but who live indoors in air-conditioning and don't get out into the sunlight may also need more of the omega 3 and 6.

Anthony Haynes, one of the UK's leading nutritional and functional medicine specialists, explained that below the neck, cell membranes work with a ratio of 4:1 of omega 6 and omega 3; hemp oil is a good supplier of oil in this ratio.

Change your diet and enjoy a good life.

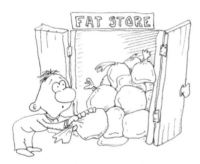

Good fat doesn't make you fat

Krebs cycle will use these short- and medium-length fatty acids to produce large numbers of ATPs, i.e. they supply our cells with energy. They have an anti-microbial and anti-fungal property in the intestines and also carry vitamins and help strengthen the immune system. They are absorbed directly through the portal vein into the liver and from there to the cells as fuel. A good source for these would be organic butter, ghee and coconut oil. These are the best for cooking as they do not turn into trans fats when heated. Look for the term unsaturated or poly-unsaturated fats—you want those.

The good, the bad and the ugly

Man-made trans or partially hydrogenated fats are produced by heating oil to very high temperatures and using a chemical solvent like nickel, resulting in a plastic-like substance. In other words, you take a healthy essential fat and 'saturate it with hydrogen' by breaking the carbon double bonds and attaching hydrogen. This is crazy and very unhealthy and is all to do with 'preserving' the shelf life of processed foods, making oils hard at room temperature and resulting in big profits through the weight loss industry. We have been sold the concept that dieting requires us to use new, low-fat spreads instead of natural butter, ghee or oils. But these low-fat spreads are dead oils, dangerous and linked to heart disease, elevated bad cholesterols, cancer and hypertension

These deadly fats are found in margarines and other low-calorie spreads as well as in crisps, biscuits and cakes found in most supermarkets. They fit into the cell membranes, but they don't work properly, so the more we eat, the less our cells can function. Remember, if a cell can't get nutrients in and waste out, it gets sick and dies. Simple solution—don't use them.

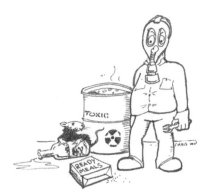

It may be too late when the chips are down.

Check all your food labels for trans fats or hydrogenated fats, and when you walk down the aisle of the supermarket, see how many rows of shelves contain dead and toxic foods. After a while you stop calling it food because it isn't. Sorry folks, that includes your chips, cookies, crisps and deep-fried foods.

Check out the dangers of canola oil (rapeseed oil), skip it and rebuild your brain and cellular health on olive oil, coconut oil, fish, hemp or cold-pressed nut oils. Kids love junk food, but do you want them to have plastic brains? Just how functional will he or she be?

No natural oils in your body means no energy! Take it easy though and don't expect miracles in a few months. You might have some good results, but I found it took me two years of a very different diet to get my energy back to the level where I have 'energy reserves'. My brain is sharp again and I can spend eight hours a day walking big mountains and skiing. It really is worth changing your diet to live a full life again!

A word of warning: beware of rancid oil—you can taste it. I was hungry one day at a small airport and gave in to the thought of chips. Against the better judgment of my inner voice, I succumbed to a bowl. Eek, after one disgusting chip the rest went in the bin. The oil had clearly not been changed in days or possibly weeks. Eating the whole bowl would have made me quite sick and would have sorely tested my liver.

Rancid oils not only found in the cooking pan. Nuts and seeds, which are predominantly fat, can go rancid with age. Being left in the air causes them to become oxidised. I've stopped buying sunflower seeds from a major high street supermarket since every time they were brown and rancid.

I also love applying oil onto my skin as a moisturiser. But again beware: often they are left on a shelf in the sun and can turn rancid, which is not nice. Don't go walking around with your face smelling of a chip shop!

> The skin is our biggest organ and our interface with the world.
> What we put on it goes straight into our blood and liver.

I try to follow the theory that if I would not ingest it, why would I put it on my skin to pollute and poison my cells? Check out your beauty lotions and potions and see if you would eat it—you probably wouldn't.

One of the key themes in this journey is detox, detox, detox. Why slap on the toxins every day and then pay a therapist to help you detox or take yourself through the unpleasant business of going through the fevers, enemas or whatever to pull them out? Crazy, huh? Ladies, I've also changed my makeup. There are some great brands out now with no parabens and free from chemicals. It's worth it, girls; let your skin radiate beauty, health and purity.

Good fats carry light into the cells

When we take in EFAs, we are giving the body the opportunity to carry light to the cells. Oils carry electron clouds in high numbers and these electrons come from the sun filling the seeds or phytoplankton with energy. They are literally 'sun foods'—light-charged electron clouds.

When the body is perfectly balanced and has enough EFAs it will naturally cope with appropriate sunlight according to its skin tone and place of birth. Always use common sense.

I have white skin and was born in northern England, so if I had all my cells made with light and healthy fats, going out for a walk would not harm me. In fact, I would be able to absorb the vitamin D and charge up my cellular batteries with photons, as well as electrons from the earth and air. However, if I was foolish enough to go for a walk without protection in Dubai, I would burn, but my dark-skinned Arab friends would not. Well, not as much. They still cover up when it gets really hot! But you get the point.

The work of Dr Johanna Budwig is worth studying for anyone interested in cellular health. An eminent German biochemist and nominated for the Nobel Peace prize seven times, she used an oil and protein protocol to successfully cure cancer. She wrote and spoke extensively on electrons and the power of EFAs to carry them. Her research studies on the blood of cancer patients versus healthy people showed that those in good health have a higher content of omega 3 than those who are sick.

She concluded that the vast presence of chronic illnesses today is due to mass-processed food and oils, poor nutrition and pesticides.

She started to treat patients and cure them with a high intake of flax oil and quark, or cottage cheese. I know it sounds whacky, but she found it cured arthritis, dissolves tumours, strengthens the heart and rescued the terminally ill. Why?

Because good oils both heal cell membranes and carry electrons. She used the cottage cheese as a high-grade protein carrier since proteins are soluble in water and can then get the oils moving more easily around the body. The amino acids that oils like best are those containing sulphur, methionine and cysteine combined with the EFAs to become lipoproteins, which are immediately available for the body to use. This is especially beneficial when the body is damaged by disease.

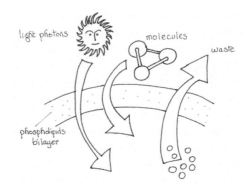

Health is movement at all levels

If you are interested in finding out more about fats, watch my interview with Antony Haynes where he shares valuable information about the correct balance of oils for both the body and the brain. He also informs us of the very successful treatment with the right kind of phospholipids and oils for healing the blood-brain barrier and Gulf War Syndrome. For more information on the blood-brain barrier and the effect of its health on various diseases, read Jeneen Interlandi's June 2013 article in Scientific American.

CHAPTER 17

Healthy Liver—Vital Life Force

After talking about getting good stuff into the body and cells, let's look at getting the toxins and waste materials out. After the cells dump their waste back into the blood stream or lymph system, it gets carried to the liver to be processed, made safe and eliminated from the body. The liver is continually processing all forms of substances from the digestive tract and the rest of your body. It is very clever and knows what can be kept and used, as well as what must leave the body. It works with two pathways: phase 1 and phase 2.

In phase 1, the liver uses enzymes to break toxins down into smaller units or raw materials, which then get shunted to phase 2. Enzymes are a kind of protein made up of long chains of different amino acids.

These phase 1 precious enzymes are susceptible to heavy metals that make them dysfunctional. This is why the removal heavy metals is a key aspect of any natural treatment for chronic diseases.

In Phase 2, these previously produced raw materials are modified by the addition of a new molecule, turning them into a new substance which is non-toxic

105

and easy to excrete. These added molecules include sulphate, methyl groups and glutathione and form three of the most important liver detoxification pathways.

Liver-based detoxification pathways are especially important for those with chronic illnesses and you may hear your therapist talking about it. The liver sulphation pathway breaks down and eliminates environmental toxins, various pharmaceutical medications and those chemicals which are produced by the body. The naturally-occurring and essential phenols and their subgroup salicylates are also targeted for elimination by this pathway. These substances need to be removed to enable effective healing.

> To maintain a good supply of enzymes to support the detoxification pathways, we need enough amino acids, which ideally come from protein in our diet.

Chronically ill Lyme patients and those with high toxicity may well require more animal protein in their diet to assist the repair and regeneration of their body.

Before I was critically ill and eaten up inside, I had been a committed vegetarian for twenty-five years, with a few of those years spent as a vegan. At one point in my healing journey, I simply had to start eating fish again. I was dreaming of eating fish and salivating each time I passed the fish counter in the supermarket. My body was shouting to me, I need animal protein! While researching and speaking with functional medicine experts in preparation for writing this chapter, it all made sense. We all need enough protein (hence, enzymes) in our diets to enable our bodies to digest well, copy DNA (make new cells), produce energy, detoxify and metabolise substances.

Liver detoxification sulphation pathway

One of the most important detoxification pathways is the sulphation pathway, which requires sulphur molecules from our diet to sustain it. Some people have a problem manufacturing sulphate and have an intolerance to sulphur-containing foods. This should be checked with your practitioner.

A large number of foods contain these toxic chemicals, with higher levels found in processed foods containing artificial flavourings, colourings and preservatives. If we ingest an unnatural excess of phenols and salicylates, we are directly taxing an important detox pathway, which is already working hard due to the illness. Whichever way we look at wellness, we inevitably keep coming back to the importance of eating healthy, fresh, organic produce in order to reduce the toxic burden on our metabolism.

Our bodies use sulphur in the form of sulphate to produce an enzyme called PST (phenol sulphurtransferase). People with Alzheimer's disease, Parkinson's disease, chemical sensitivities and rheumatoid arthritis are often shown to have a reduced ability to produce enough sulphates.

Lyme is called the great imitator and causes memory loss like Alzheimer's, neurological problems akin to Parkinson's and frequently causes arthritic symptoms.

It may be that as this detox pathway becomes overburdened and phenols start backing up, some of these Lyme symptoms emerge.

Sulphur can enter our body through both nutrition and the skin. My two easy-to-use favourites are the supplement MSM (methylsulfonylmethane) and for transdermal absorption Epsom salts (magnesium sulphate). Bathing in Epsom salts is a very old, natural remedy with double benefit, as you get both sulphur and magnesium. Borrelia has been shown to reduce magnesium levels in almost all Lyme patients, making Epsom salts a valuable, cheap and effective tool in recovery.

In Epsom salts, the sulphur is in the form of a sulphate ion, which is immediately available for use and does not need to be converted. Should you be lucky enough to live near some natural hot springs where the water is rich in minerals and sulphur, you would benefit greatly from a weekly soak!

To use Epsom salts, simply add a cup or two to a lovely warm bath and lie back for twenty minutes and soak. If you don't have a bath, simply soak your feet or hands in a basin of warm water containing Epsom salts and the minerals will be absorbed directly through the skin. Some people like to make up a cream and rub the salt on the skin and others like to spray it on your skin, but this can cause some dryness. After a bath or foot soak, if your skin feels dry, apply some natural body oil or coconut oil to moisturise.

Digging into the sulphur story

Earlier in the sulphation section, I mentioned the need for MSM (Methylsulfonylmethane), the naturally occurring sulphur that is biologically active and is found in all living organisms from enzymes and tissues to hormones and antioxidants. It is the third most abundant element in life on earth and MSM is 34 percent elemental sulphur by weight, making it one of the richest sources of sulphur we can ingest.

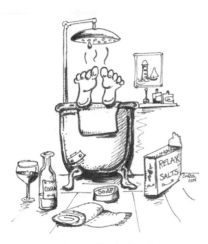

…then add a little salt!

In my own journey to health after the ravages of Lyme disease, it has been one of my key health recovery factors. Interestingly, one of my less painful but annoying complaints after a decade of Lyme disease was a terrible nail complaint. My finger nails would split and flake and crack and I always carry around a nail file as there is nothing more annoying than split nails scratching and catching on all your clothes and tights. That's not important per se, but, as with all symptoms, it points back to a need to change something, i.e., to make the nail protein, 'keratin', stronger.

Along these lines, my hair started to come out in handfuls in the shower and hair is also made of keratin. Sulphur may well be the missing link, as it is part of the connective tissue protein collagen, which literally runs through the whole body and helps keep the tissues elastic and flexible. Collagen, in turn, helps form cartilage.

I also wonder whether this could also have been a contributing factor in my muscle and joint dryness. One day the spring literally went out of my step. Jumping and landing were painful, and my body felt old and dried out. Once I started taking MSM, my nails improved for good, my hair is back to being a thick mop, my joints and muscles are no longer sore and dry and that spring and bounce is back when I exercise.

When choosing your MSM, check that it has trace amounts of molybdenum as this is needed for sulphur to be effective.

If the MSM you choose does not have this added, your body will have to use its own stores, causing more problems. This trace element has numerous roles, including activating enzymes associated with antioxidants, digestion of foods, creating new cells, etc. It also has a role to play in metabolising toxins, drugs and generally helping the body eliminate waste.

Why is our diet not enough?

Sulphur is part of the detoxification pathways of the cells and my body was swimming in toxins, as we have seen already. It works to make the cell wall more permeable, which in turn will allow the toxins out and nutrients in. The sulphur molecule also binds to the toxin, which neutralises it, and given that the Borrelia was everywhere and creating neurotoxins in unreasonable quantities, the body would soon be running out of its sulphur supplies. The body is very clever and whenever it needs something and can't get a fresh supply, it will take it from less important areas like nails and hair to do its crucial work.

The other benefit of MSM is the methyl group (CH3), which is used by the body in many important biochemical processes that rely on methylation, including the metabolism of lipids and DNA. In essence, methylation is needed for the construction and destruction processes of the cells. Given the crucial importance of methylation it seems likely that MSM will be a very useful supplement for many conditions, including depression and ageing given that the body's ability to methylate declines with age.

MSM occurs naturally in the oceans, rain water and in the food chain; however, we are not living in that perfect, organic, unadulterated world, so it can easily be deficient in our diets. Ed McCabe, in his book Flood Your Body with Oxygen, explains the intricate pathway from oceanic soup to our food chain. In the ocean, a sea of minerals and oxygen, plankton produce oxygen and sulphur compounds called dimethylsulphonium salts. These become dimethylesulphide (DMS) in the sea water and then evaporate into the air and clouds collide with ozone and UV light to be converted into MSM and DMSO (dimethyl sulfoxide), which falls back to earth in raindrops to be taken up by fruit and vegetable plants, grasses, etc.

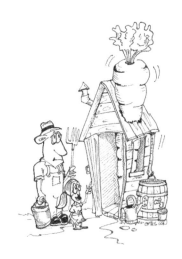

Hence, when we eat our raw, organic, rain-fed vegetables, we are starting to give our body a reasonable supply of sulphur in a safe and natural way. In the wild, certain plants absorb more MSM, such as pine bark, needles and nuts, wild grasses, noni fruit and aloe vera. MSM is extracted from these plants and is available in supplemental

Too much organic seaweed Dad!

crystal powder form. When purchasing MSM, it is important to ensure that it has a degree of purity of over 99.99 percent. It should also be derived from pine trees, but unfortunately some manufacturers extract it from petrochemicals, so beware! Also beware, don't eat uncooked or undercooked beans which contain high amounts of glycoprotein lectin, a toxin that can cause nausea, vomiting and diarrhea within three hours of consumption. Potato can also have a similar effect if eaten raw.

In my grandfather's garden, he always had wooden barrels of rainwater collected from the greenhouse and potting shed roof. His entire garden was watered by this rainwater and one of my treats as a wee nipper was to go into the greenhouse and eat the baby tomatoes. I can still remember their smell and taste to this day and only on a few occasions, with a very special organic garden, do I find anything comparable. Nowadays, very little of our agriculture is irrigated by rainwater. It's mostly not organic and unfortunately much of our soil is demineralised.

Various scientists are finding ways to re-mineralise our earth and I feel it's worth a mention here for all you gardeners, organic buffs and farmers aiming for higher yields to explore if you haven't already done so. David Wolfe, in one of his talks, explains how he gives pure seawater to his plants on his farm in Hawaii.

The use of seaweed as fertiliser has been used for generations to help enrich the soil with minerals from the sea.

I grew up in Scotland and was familiar with the Findhorn community, where huge vegetables were grown in very poor soil. Some of this was said to be due to the founder's ability to talk to Devas of the vegetable kingdom and some may well have been due to good fertiliser and volcanic rock dust.

Master supplement matters

MSM has so many benefits. Let's explore a few more, just so you get the picture!

- It helps in the repair of tissue damage, aids in mobility and increases flexibility.
- In sports, it reduces the build-up of lactic acid and, therefore, cramps.
- MSM helps oxygenate the blood and thus the body, which in turn deters the growth of bacteria, fungus and viruses.
- Sulphur is a component of insulin and some cases of diabetes and hypoglycaemia have been associated with low sulphur levels.
- The increase in cell permeability aids the absorption of nutrients and oxygen into the cells along with the release of toxins, thereby helping to increase energy levels.
- Reduces inflammation and swelling by helping the cells flush out toxins.

- Helps alleviate skin, nail and hair conditions.
- Topical application of MSM has been shown to help wounds heal quickly without scarring.

Taking a low concentration of MSM is being associated with reducing the effects of stress, both physiological and physical, organ and tissue malfunction and fatigue and susceptibility to disease. There are a number of studies done with osteoarthritis showing that bathing in sulphurous water reduces pain, stiffness and improves quality of life. Other studies show that arthritic cartilage contains up to one third less sulphur than healthy cartilage.

Sulphur is an integral part of two main amino acids in the body: methionine and cysteine. AIDS sufferers show a deviation from the normal composition of the body's amino acid pool in that they have a marked shortage of these same amino acids. Dr. Johanna Budwig's research into helping cancer patients and curing other diseases stresses that the favourable oils used for healthy cell membranes require these two sulphur-based amino acids.

We are just beginning to realise how and why sulphur is so important and why it is the sixth most abundant macro-mineral in breast milk and the third most abundant mineral based on percentage of total body weight.

Beat the hangovers!

Sulphur is also reported to be able to normalise certain body functions in patients displaying gastrointestinal upset, inflammation of mucus membranes, allergic reactions, drug hypersensitivity and inflammatory disorders, including arthritis, muscle cramps and infectious parasites. MSM is also said to control acidity in the stomach, which may be useful in cases of ulcers. Various testimonials indicate that MSM is particularly beneficial in cases of emphysema, allergies, candida, diabetes, diverticulitis, chronic headaches, hypoglycaemia, Alzheimer's disease, athlete's foot and hangovers!

With a list like that, it's worth giving it a try and, like so many of these great gifts of nature, to date there are no known toxic effects from MSM. However, it is best to start taking MSM in small quantities. Initially I started with ¼ tablespoon in ½ litre of water and increased the dose gradually to one to two tablespoons each day. Don't do what I did due to a very hectic international travel schedule and stop taking your MSM. Thinking 'I'd better catch up,' I immediately put two tablespoons in a glass of water and gulped it back. The next day my face was covered in white pimples containing pus. The sulphur was kicking out toxins at too fast a rate for my liver and normal detox pathways and the skin, our biggest organ, pushed them out to remedy the situation. For a week, I felt rather embarrassed walking around looking like someone with a plague in a horror movie.

The message is clear: taking it slowly and easing the dosage up over weeks and months makes MSM a great aid. Other ways to increase or maintain sulphur levels in the body are by eating the relevant foods and taking superfoods like spirulina, bee pollen, macca, noni juice and marine phytoplankton. The first three are always in my morning super smoothie. Sulphur rich foods would include broccoli, garlic, kale, onions and radishes. MSM is denatured by heating and food processing, so ensure you either take the crystal powder or eat some raw organic veggies every day. It is considered extremely safe and does not produce toxic waste in the body.

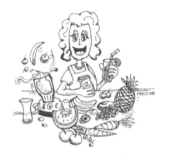

The lesson I took away from the 'spotty face' experience is the reminder never to suddenly jump in and blast one's body with a massive dose of something without first thinking it through, or checking with your therapist, and always starting with low doses! 'Patience' is not my middle name,

Don't smother yourself on smoothies too quickly

but this healing journey is making me learn the art of building foundations, slowly and surely. Many times, therapists have discussed with me their understanding of holistic healing protocols. What becomes apparent is that the length of time we have abused our bodies should be considered. The longer we have taken drugs for various symptoms, ignored the warning signs, overridden its cries for help or been overrun by microbes will determine how long recovery will take.

> It may take two years for your body to be rebuilt and fully well again after a serious illness.

The longer we do those destructive things, the longer it will take to repair and rebuild. If it's been out of kilter for a decade or more, it can't suddenly find perfect health, vitality and harmony overnight. Much has to change within us as composite body, mind, emotional and spiritual beings to find perfect synergy once again. An imbalance in our biochemistry not only affects the physical body, but also our mind and emotions. Holistic practitioners and functional medicine doctors monitor and assist all aspects of our health picture.

CHAPTER 18

Removing Toxins and Chemicals

Methylation is crucial in the breakdown and removal of toxins and hormones. In particular, it targets: natural oestrogens, phytoestrogens (chemical copies) and xenobiotics (those multiple toxic chemicals found in our air, water, food chain, houses, offices, factories and schools).

It converts toxins of all kinds from insoluble, less soluble or fat-soluble compounds into water-soluble compounds (often by adding a CH3 group). This in turn allows the body to eliminate them more easily.

Methylation is found throughout the body, playing a key role in the manufacture and breakdown of various neurotransmitters, including adrenaline (epinephrine) and melatonin. As methylation plays so many crucial roles, anyone with a chronic disease, especially Lyme, should check and support its efficacy.

Many of the side effects of Lyme disease may stem from poor methylation. The addition or removal of the Methyl (CH3) group is solely dependent on ATP (your body's preferred energy source). Those ATP molecules that are used for methylation must be attached to a magnesium molecule for the ATP to work.

Detoxifying the body needs time, otherwise you stress your organs and deplete valuable enzyme supplies.

Borrelia competes for magnesium, which it uses for building biofilms. This lowers the available magnesium and, therefore, methylation potential. Many Lyme practitioners often need to recommend magnesium supplementation. However, please check if you need it and in what form. It can be taken orally or via the skin as a cream or oil. I personally have found magnesium citrate tablets to be the most effective and still carry them should I get a cramp, and they also stop me from getting altitude sickness while skiing in the Alps. Alcohol is contraindicated with Lyme disease, as it closes down methylation pathways and uses up Glutathione stores! Sorry folks, it's time to abstain until you are back to full health.

Still interested in the methylation business?

The methylation process first tags dangerous substances and then alters them in such a way that the body can identify them as toxins, after which they are ready to be eliminated quickly. Larger molecules are eliminated through the bile, while smaller ones pass into the bloodstream and are removed by the kidneys in the urine. Have you noticed that naturopathic therapists are concerned with how much you poo and pee as well as when and what it looks and smells like? This is for a very good reason, because the practitioner needs to know how well our elimination pathways are operating—whether they're open and healthy.

There is a lot more to methylation worth mentioning and for those who are ill it is especially important. It is part of the synthesis and utilisation of neurotransmitters called dopamine and serotonin. Disrupted sleep patterns and mood swings are all part of the large bag of Lyme symptoms and increasing magnesium and hence methylation may help with those two conditions.

Methylation is a key step in the formation of our enzymes and proteins. This process is called genetic transcription and first involves making a copy of a section of DNA, which is a strand of RNA. This is the blueprint for our proteins, which the body uses to put together the exact proteins that are needed.

Yes, even anti-ageing needs methylation, which is involved in the preservation of the body's 'tails' (telomeres) on its DNA and chromosomes. The 'tails' shorten and lessen in number with age, so if you want to look good, feel great and grow old with dignity and adventure, keep your methylation pathways up and running! Whatever our age, diet choices or health status, we need more methyl groups. No one can avoid all stress and toxins, but we can bring awareness to supporting ourselves with correct daily choices.

Increase your methyl groups

Your body is already producing methyl groups naturally, and a healthy diet will provide a good source of methyl groups through lamb, chicken, beets, quinoa, spinach and generally lots of lightly-cooked, dark green veggies. Raw food is not the ideal diet in this case, and avoid microwave and processed foods. Vegetarians may need to supplement with TMG (Trimethylglycine) after checking with their health practitioner.

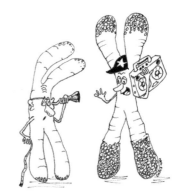

Sugar is a no-no; it does not help methylation and fermented food intake should be limited. Moderation is key in consuming kefir, yogurt, miso and good quality cheese as these do not use up essential methyl groups.

Dude, you must be on Methylation!

Some supplements containing zinc, magnesium, copper, calcium and other minerals help the production of methyl groups. Your practitioner may also recommend you take folate (especially in the form of 5 methyltetrahydrofolate), B6 (in the active form of P5P) and B12 (in the active form of methylcobalamin).

CHAPTER 19

Your Master Antioxidant

Glutathione (or GSH) is our ultimate friend and one of the most important molecules in the body to mention in the quest for good health. Our ability to produce and maintain a high level of Glutathione is critical to prevent disease, recover from Lyme and other chronic illnesses, boost energy levels and maintain peak performance. Glutathione is a protein molecule made by the body and found in every cell. It consists of three amino acids: cysteine, glutamate and glycine. It is the most powerful of antioxidants and is made in our immune cells, where it enhances activity.

Glutathione has multiple functions, including detoxifying at cellular levels and regulating cell growth and division. It repairs and aids cells and DNA synthesis by donating electrons. In a healthy cell, we have enough Glutathione standing by to donate. However, if we have used up our supply of GSH and therefore have no readily available free electrons, a chain reaction can set in.

The problem is that once a molecule loses its electron, it too becomes a free radical and wants to steal from others nearby. If not balanced by antioxidants donating free electrons, this chain reaction can lead to cell death or DNA mutilation.

If we run out of Glutathione, we are not able to protect ourselves from all kinds of cancer, infections and free radicals.

In the liver, the enzyme Glutathione S-transferase takes the sulphur from Glutathione and attaches it to toxic molecules, making the toxins more water-soluble. In this state, it can be more easily eliminated from the body via the usual pathways. This is another reason to stay very hydrated when doing any kind of detox and working with Herx or healing reactions. If we don't drink enough quality, clean water, the body will end up reabsorbing the toxins and counteracting all your good work!

Glutathione contains that wonderful ingredient, sulphur, which creates a glue-like component that attracts toxins, heavy metals and free radicals to it. In turn, these can be safely eliminated from the body. Glutamate and glycine are readily available in a healthy diet, but to get cysteine we need to make more effort as it tends to get broken down and altered before reaching cellular levels.

Our ancestors had a ready supply through consumption of raw milk, cheese and yogurt, but modern, pasteurised dairy doesn't help us as the amino acid is denatured during the enormous heating process.

It is hard to find fresh, raw milk products, so an alternative would be to add a daily measure of organic, grass fed, raw, totally pure whey powder to your diet. Ensure it is bioactive and made from non-denatured proteins.

So, what leads to lowered Glutathione levels?

Many factors use our supply of GSH for neutralising and detoxifying and like the proverbial camel and his load, we can't say which one leads to a critical point, but all should be addressed, including: poor diet, pollution, stress, toxins, industrial chemicals, herbicides, pesticides, heavy metals (especially mercury and lead) drugs and medications, trauma, ageing, e-smog, radiation, as well as multiple viral, parasitic or bacterial infections. As you can see, that list includes pretty much all the things mentioned in this book that need to be addressed in order to recover from chronic illness.

Looking at that list, we ought to think about our genes. Are we biologically geared to survive such an onslaught of man-made toxins? The answer is NO. Only about 50 percent of the population have the genetic capacity—the GSTM1 function—required in the process of effectively creating and recycling Glutathione in the body. Mark Hyman, a functional medicine doctor in the US, says, 'Nearly all my very sick patients are missing this function.'

This is a worrying discovery and may suggest that testing becomes essential for people with chronic illnesses.

The ratio of reduced Glutathione (GSH) to oxidised Glutathione (GSSG) within cells can be used as a measure of cellular toxicity. I would like to see these tests cheaply available for everyone to use on a yearly basis, like getting your car checked. To be healthy we need more than 90 percent of the reduced form (GSH) in each cell.

Would dinosaurs survive now?

Probably not! Only in the last seventy years or so has mankind been heavily throwing horrible chemicals into the food chain, water supplies and lotions and potions. Before that, most people ate organic, fresh food, home-made, in season and usually locally sourced. It's all gotten out of hand. Preserved foods used to be naturally made by pickling with vinegar, using sugar syrups or drying and fermenting (as in wine or beer).

In fact, my mother still makes jams, chutneys, wine and other delicious preserves made from local fruit and vegetables.

Thousands of years ago, as humanity evolved, no one needed a massive chemical and e-smog detox programme in our DNA. Hence, there was no need for this

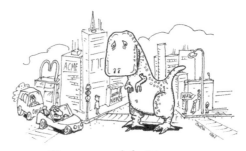

Times are tough for Dinosaurs

aspect of our DNA programming to develop as a primary survival tool. More and more people today are struggling with various health problems stemming from a reaction to the sea of chemicals we now live in.

> Who knows how long it will take for humans to adapt to living in this highly-polluted world? We have messed up our nest and now we must live with the repercussions both short-term (our life now) and long-term (generational). Making your diet and environment as unpolluted as possible is key to surviving and thriving in the coming decades.

Glutathione in a nutshell

1. Every cell needs Glutathione (GSH) to be healthy and energised.

2. If GSH is used for neutralising toxins, it is not as available to do its main job of restoring wellness.

3. We are losing large amounts of GSH through elimination with the toxins we need to replace it.

4. Let's stop the rot, prevent further wastage or future ill health by cleaning up our internal and external habitat. In turn, this will protect the most valuable asset we have against disease and ageing.

There are over 100,000 medical research papers on Glutathione and it has been clinically proven that by raising your GSH level, your health will benefit in multiple ways. Young or old, athletic or infirm, we all benefit from optimising our Glutathione levels. The mitochondria of a cell require Glutathione to remain fully charged, thus enhancing vitality, muscle strength and endurance. Clinical trials have shown that lowering GSH in the mitochondria results in cell death.

Just some of the conditions which have benefited from increasing GSH levels include: Alzheimer's, asthma, burns, cancer, chronic fatigue syndrome, diabetes, autoimmune disorders, diseases of liver, kidneys, lungs, heart, the digestive system, flu, fibromyalgia, hepatitis, multiple sclerosis, Parkinson's, physical trauma, skin disorders, seizures, tumours and more.

Are you getting excited about Glutathione?

It also has many other functions, including immunity, which is involved in protein synthesis and amino acid transport both in and out of cells and between them. Immune system function is especially dependent on GSH.

A bit about enzymes: Glutathione acts like a bridge to activate and catalyse the chemical reaction between some enzymes and is the mechanism by which many enzymes are reduced, transformed or changed from one state to another.

On the negative side, Xenobiotics is an exotic-sounding word for rather nasty substances: those chemical components which are unnatural or foreign to the body, such as drugs, food additives and environmental pollutants. Glutathione is a scavenger and will grab the oxidised baddies cell by cell.

Quite often a chronic illness or fatigue problem begins with an extreme toxic load.

One example of this is caused by the removal of amalgam fillings. Many people today have mercury fillings that were taken out after realising they were slowly poisoning themselves. However, very few dentists do this with impeccable care using specialised equipment, gum shields, masks and air filters to ensure you don't inhale or swallow the mercury as it is removed.

I experienced this myself when I had three mercury fillings removed in one sitting by a regular dentist and within six months started experiencing serious health problems. Glutathione is an invaluable friend, as it will bond to mercury and other heavy metals, neutralising them and eliminating them from the body.

For frequent fliers, a rare but worrying toxicity is the chance of hydraulic fuel, jet oil and other toxic engine fumes, including organophosphates, escaping into the cabin. It only takes a trace amount of those fumes to cause a toxic reaction in the body. There are numerous cases of airline staff suffering from chronic fatigue, memory loss, headaches, digestive problems, dizziness and many other symptoms. We will all keep flying, of course, but it's just another reason to keep ahead of the detox game and support our antioxidants and boost detox pathways.

A bit about radiation: Glutathione also detoxifies reactive oxygen radicals created by radiation and UV radiation damage; this reduces the damage to the cell. With all the

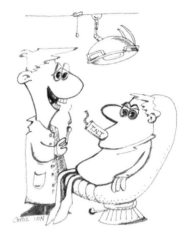

Mercury looks better in the sky.

nuclear power station accidents and leaks in the past fifty years, I have a suspicion this particular problem will become a major player in the detox game in the years to come.

A very interesting theory proposed by Rich Van Konynenburg Ph.D. explores the link between Borrelia and our depletion of Glutathione. In short, he explains that Borrelia requires cysteine for its metabolism, which it absorbs directly from the body and uses to produce its own essential enzymes and support its survival. By reducing cysteine, we reduce our levels of Glutathione.

He goes on to make a further suggestion that when we have lowered Glutathione and low Glutathione peroxidase activity, our hydrogen peroxide concentration and cellular oxidative stress increases. This, he suggests, allows Borrelia to turn into its cyst form, which is more difficult for the body or antibiotics to destroy.

> What is clear is that Borrelia requires cysteine, and, in taking what it wants, it robs us of our master antioxidant.

The big boss

In her book, Stop Aging Now!, Jean Carper claims, 'You must get your levels of GSH up if you want to keep your youth and live longer. High levels of GSH predict good health and long life. Low levels predict early disease and death.'

> Lowered Glutathione = Increased Fatigue

Glutathione plays the role of the master antioxidant to recycle oxidised lipoic acid, as well as vitamins C and E, by restoring them to an active state, mostly by donating the electrons that they used in metabolising free radicals. This means they are not eliminated from the body, which would mean hard work for the cells to make new ones. This is one good reason to look into your Vitamin C and E intake and supplements.

And, finally, a natural approach to increasing Glutathione is via the use of turmeric. This ancient spice contains curcumin, which has been used medically in Asian countries for centuries. It has anti-inflammatory, antioxidant, anti-cancer and neuroprotective activities. When curcumin is used with piperine (an extract of black pepper) it works even more effectively. The Linus Pauling Institute explains, 'In the test tube, curcumin has been shown as an effective scavenger of reactive oxygen species (ROS) and reactive nitrogen species.'

It is also being researched for its ability to 'induce the expression of phase II antioxidant enzymes, including glutamate-cysteine ligase (GCL) the rate-limiting enzyme in Glutathione synthesis.'

I personally take specific turmeric supplements from Japan, as well as enjoy cooking with the powder or fresh root as often as possible. My health increased noticeably with this particular product, with inflammation down and energy up!

In the book Glutathione. Your Body's Most Powerful Protector, Dr. Jimmy Gutman says, 'Glutathione modulation is an essential part of staying young, active and healthy. By keeping our intracellular GSH levels up we also keep our immune system on the ball and fully armed.'

Some practitioners will test you and suggest increasing cysteine levels by administering oral N-acetylcysteine (NAC), which is then converted into circulating cysteine for Glutathione synthesis. Another approach for supplementation is that of taking activated B12 (methylcobalamin), which is a precursor of methionine, which in turn is a precursor of cysteine and hence ultimately Glutathione. Selenium has been shown to help the body recycle Glutathione, but, as always, you need to be tested and monitored before taking supplements; never self-diagnose.

Your daily diet should contain sulphur-rich foods. These include: garlic, onions, broccoli, kale, collards, cabbage, cauliflower and watercress.

Ensure you are eating well and making fresh food for yourself each day. Leftovers and packaged foods have little or no nutrients.

It can be hard when you are exhausted with Lyme and other diseases, but eating well is crucial to getting better. Exercise is also part of building Glutathione levels and you can't beat a thirty-minute brisk walk in nature.

Whatever you enjoy, do it and move the body. If you are at the chronic stage of any disease and living with exhaustion (I know what that's like and you are not alone), I recommend my Beyond Fatigue online movement course which is designed and made for people in or recovering from illnesses and chronic fatigue of any kind. It will help you get moving without crashing, stimulate your immune system and help lymphatic drainage.

In short, help yourself and become your very own Glutathione guardian and watch your health and immunity soar.

CHAPTER 20

Health Care is Going to Change

Although there are no quick fixes to keep a healthy and vibrant body, there are ways you can take care of yourself and, bit by bit, you will notice a difference in how you feel.

It doesn't have to be hard work; in fact, it can be fun and sociable.

The key is to plan ahead and stay well so you don't reach out for strong medication at the smallest sniffle. We need to put aside strong drugs like antibiotics and only use them when they are desperately needed.

Instead, we need to explore natural anti-pain and anti-inflammatory treatments, many of which have been used for generations.

They may not have been subjected to double-blind controlled trials, but they have been used for so long that the proof lies simply in their repeated results. Have you tried Chinese or Ayurvedic medicine? What about ozone, herbs, homeopathy, massage, yoga therapy, naturopathy and so on. Explore and ask others and the right solutions or therapies will come your way. Taking a sauna once a week is great for detoxing and provides time to relax, unwind, connect with friends at the spa and so on.

I have had two great health retreats at Ayurvedic health centres in Southern India, where I was cared for by super staff and doctors who really know their stuff. To become an Ayurvedic Physician in India, you have to first complete a full regular medical degree that takes over five years before starting your six-year Ayurvedic medical studies. That's some dedication and knowledge base. I enjoyed the massages, and although some of the five-stage Panchakarma treatments were intense, they were effective.

> We live in uncertain and exciting times that require a different way of thinking.

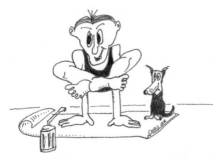

Create your own new-look lifestyle

I believe medical tourism will become the norm in the years to come. People who can't get the treatments they want in one country will travel around the world to enterprising retreat centres or small hotels in beautiful, natural locations. Here they will be cared for by dedicated teams of health specialists, along with some Frequency and Bioenergy devices, fresh air, clean water, wild earth and great nutrition. The old concept of sanatoriums will return with a whole new mission and outlook.

CHAPTER 21

The Mind, Body Conundrum

We exist as an entire organism comprised of the body, mind, soul, emotions, genes, molecules, ions, meridians, memories and more. Every part of us, visible and invisible, is controlled, organised, repaired or removed by a coherent, quantum, electrodynamic field.

Quantum coherence ensures we just can't get away from this beautiful concept of wholeness and this living, intelligent field of information which enables each molecule to communicate with all the others, apparently simultaneously.

If we are doing everything in this book, and maybe more, to care for ourselves, yet still feel unwell or unhappy, what else could be going wrong?

The missing link lies with our mind, our consciousness, our ego structure and personality, all of which play a lead role in changing both our energy and our physical reality.

Quantum entanglement explains what the ancient mystics said: 'know yourself and you know the universe'. It also follows that what we do to ourselves, we do to others, including the earth itself, for good or bad. When you change inner attitudes, becoming truly content, you heal yourself. This is not about those transitory moments of happiness experienced when we acquire a new job, dress or car, but rather the deep heartfelt contentment gained from living in harmony with yourself and your world.

> Feeling loved or happy deep in your heart will send out a message of peace and wholeness to ricochet across the galaxy, influencing all beings.

The search for meaning, purpose and wholeness is just as old as mankind. Many teachers have led the way and found unconditional love. This awakened state is also called freedom or Oneness, because you have freed yourself from carrying negative thoughts and emotions; thus, allowing you to see the higher purpose of all things. You live with congruence and in awareness of your connection to all of the unlimited energy field behind creation.

As such, your feelings, thoughts, words and actions are like a single musical note. In that moment, they sing the same transparent and empowering message. This state is the immortal cup that so many seek. In such a state, the body is not decaying; it is being recharged and rejuvenated with creativity, harmony and joy.

The vast majority of people live disconnected from this truth. They may think one thing yet say something else, and their hearts have yet another desire or need. Healing is also bringing us back to this state of coherence. Imagine the confused frequencies and wave patterns your immune system must be getting if you keep carrying deep-seated feelings of hate, fear, greed or envy?

So, along with the physical and electrical toxicity mankind has created on earth, we are also subjecting our bodies to these damaging thoughts and feelings.

When we look at all life as sitting within a quantum coherent universe, every part of us is both here as a solid object (or particle) and simultaneously delocalised as quantum wave functions. This means we are literally everywhere in this moment and entangled with everyone else's 'presence', which is also everywhere.

This concept—our interconnection with all things—could be one of the greatest mysteries of life, waiting for each of us to explore.

> The discovery of our entanglement and the responsibility that lies inherent within this knowledge must be the next step for humanity if we are to survive as a species.

What a beautiful realisation—I am an infinite being, reaching out across creation, in constant communication with all beings. And most importantly, I am the captain of my own ship. With knowledge comes responsibility. Knowing photons and electrons are essential for vitality, we can now take every opportunity to get out into nature. Understanding how cells work will hopefully entice us to choose to protect them from free radicals. These are just two little ideas that, when followed through, will radically change our lives for the better.

Taking time through meditation, contemplation or reflection is an age-old technique to help us take charge of our emotional maturity and attitude towards life. Regardless of past difficulties, you can choose right now to change your perception, adopt new value systems and dance to a more beautiful tune. I often say to my coaching clients: 'are you in control of your mind or is your mind in control of you?' We want to be in charge of ourselves, not just so we can aid healing, but also to achieve our dreams and goals, do our jobs well and use each day wisely. One second of a positive thought or emotion will instantly (faster than the speed of light) cause neurons to fire to relax a muscle, release enzymes or move electrons to heal a site of inflammation or trauma.

On a day-to-day basis, just how do we change these mental and emotional patterns?

What if...

Let's play a game for a moment called 'What if...?'

What if I got this illness/problem/challenge for a higher purpose?

For example, 'Instead of ignoring my body, diet, stress levels etc.', you could say to yourself: 'I will use my suffering as a wake-up call and make irrevocable good health choices from now on. I know that it is not just for my own benefit, but for that of my loved ones and those suffering elsewhere'. Or you could think along the lines of 'what did I do to get myself into this pickle?' Did I argue a lot? Stress over money? Ignore signs of fatigue? Take too many chemical drugs (legal or otherwise)? And so on.

Another way to explore the bigger picture is to detach yourself from the physical, mental and emotional pain and simply watch. Inside of you is your immortal Spirit; it does not have a disease. It is the seat of your higher self, your awareness with unlimited power; it is the indwelling witness of all that is. Let this part of you shine out like a light and focus on it.

Remember, what you focus on grows. It's all too easy to bemoan your lot, but it takes real courage to keep your mind focused on the higher truth. This exercise strengthens our willpower and reconnects us to the source field, which supplies all information and energy. For those with faith in a Divine or God, this approach brings you closer to feeling connected with that Power.

What if your pain and suffering are here to bring you closer to your undiluted self, the part of you that is free, happy and uncluttered?

This is the truth, but most of us have spent our lives associating with our need for physical comfort and emotional support. We are told by marketing companies that our happiness lies in obtaining another dress, a new car, a big wedding or some special shampoo that will make us more beautiful. Sorry folks, but that's a pile of old rubbish! If you have been through some level of intense suffering, I'm sure that you have realised happiness lies in a moment when you are at peace. When a friend smiles at you and shares a joke, or when you sit and watch a butterfly alight upon a delicate bloom in the garden.

When you are deeply in pain, or even in one of those dark nights of the soul, does another pair of shiny shoes pull you up? No, of course not! Does the thought of buying a new car or bigger house make you dance? No! In fact, you don't want the hassle of more material possessions. How much energy will it take to look after it, clean it, deal with the paperwork and so on? When we are at the end of our tether of life expectancy, we start to make a new priority list and view life quite differently. Why wait to be pulled down to this extreme level of disharmony before changing the way we see life? Do it now!

Once you accept where you are, without judgment or condemnation of yourself or others, you can make a plan and start moving forward, changing your frequency and cellular health patterns.

Don't linger in the past either—you have no strength there.

In fact, looking back only dilutes your energy. It's one of the greatest ways to leak life-force. There's nothing we can do about what has been—it's done and gone. Yet many people spend a great deal of time dwelling on past pain, disappointments and difficulties. If you must think of the past, think of joyful and empowering moments that bring you strength. Beware of falling into denial or in an aggressive mode where you are diluting life force, our precious energy, away from the healing that needs to happen.

Enlightened and empowered

The less energy you have, the more you will inevitably cut down on the non-essentials of life. All pain is a wake-up call, and, if used well, will become the greatest tool for your heroic spiritual awakening. You don't have to go to a church or temple to find God and gain enlightened, empowered moments. They usually happen when you least expect them, in moments of intense surrender and acceptance.

I do however believe in the power of coming together in silent communion, meditation or prayer. Ask people to pray for you if you are unwell—even if you're not a believer in God. The power of intention is massive, and when positive people gather to focus on sending you light, energy and hope, it works. Remain open-minded. You never know what miracles are just around the corner.

> Any life-threatening illness or extremely stressful life event prompts us to reflect on what really matters.

Often due to past, personal or social traumas, we block our minds from seeing possible answers from the Universe (answers to our prayers, and so on). If we shut down and become negative, we may miss an offer of help from an unexpected source or be unwilling to try a different source of healing. We may shut out loved ones or a stranger's kind words. In essence, stay open to all the gifts of change, light and possibility that will come to you as you journey to your ultimate freedom.

We all need to be part of a community or group of friends; these are essential for our emotional and psychological wellness. There are very few people who feel they can exist in isolation. We are hard-wired to feel and give love, help others and enjoy social interaction. If you are feeling isolated, remember that frequency is being broadcast to your holographic and molecular body, which in turn will be thrown into disharmony. Temporarily, this should not cause a problem as your whole self will work to bring back homeostasis and the natural order of interconnection. But if you carry this feeling intensely and for long periods of time, it will eventually impact one or more aspects of yourself. Healing must include feelings, beliefs and attitudes if it is to be completely effective.

The mystic schools of the East say that we are not the body, but that we are great beings of light with a human incarnation. I love that! We can but endeavour to steer our lives away from fragmentation and illness towards greater contentment and healing. Let's work together to explore and live our wildest dreams and embrace this ancient (although new to some) paradigm of Frequency and Bioenergy.

Conclusion

As a species, we have taken one huge leap of what we thought was progress, but instead it has led to disaster on all planes of existence. We moved away from nature into concrete cities. In doing so, humanity is gradually losing its connection to the source of all life, and with it, the access to a higher and more spiritual energy field. Healing humanity and the planet will require all of us to reconnect to light and energy. The simplest way to do that is to spend time in nature. Harmonise your frequencies in all ways, from thoughts to reducing Wi-Fi exposure. In brief, detoxify your cells, your environment and your life!

> Healing humanity and the planet will require all of us to reconnect with light and energy.

Cook good food, share and eat it with others. Return to good, old-fashioned values like love, respect and kindness; these are the golden threads uniting you with all others. In the end, it is the simple things that matter and make us well.

Our modern lives have taken mankind far from this simple but powerful connection to the source. So far, in fact, that most people have forgotten where we came from. Mother Earth and the Sun have enormous power. Let light heal you and the raw power of nature fill your cells!

Meanwhile, the truth is that technological advances are here to stay. We won't and can't just give them up and go 'off the grid'. Progress means moving forwards, not backwards, and there is much to be done by all of us to redirect our science and wisdom to serve us, not destroy us.

The era of the superbug is also upon us, and Antimicrobial Resistance (AMR) is an ever-growing global threat. The World Health Organization (WHO) calls for all countries to implement an action plan and states that 'single, isolated interventions have limited impact. Coordinated action is required to minimise the emergence and spread of antimicrobial resistance.'

I believe that now is the time for international exploration and implementation of Frequency and Bioenergy medicine as a cost-effective and practical aspect of daily healthcare. The newer drugs being developed by big pharma have serious side-effects—will this be your choice? Already, 12,000 people in the UK alone die of antibiotic-resistant superbugs each year. That's more than breast cancer. If we don't embrace Frequency and Bioenergy methods, start promoting and protecting natural (and ancient) forms of healthcare and change our approach to nutrition, we can look ahead to a future in which people die from simple cuts and infections. This is predicted to happen by 2050.

In May 2016, The Review on Antimicrobial Resistance (AMR), chaired by Jim O'Neill, stated:

> "The magnitude of the problem is now accepted. We estimate that by 2050, 10 million lives a year and a cumulative 100 trillion USD of economic output are at risk due to the rise of drug-resistant infections if we do not find proactive solutions now to slow down the rise of drug resistance. Even today, 700,000 people die of resistant infections every year. Antibiotics are a special category of antimicrobial drugs that underpin modern medicine as we know it: if they lose their effectiveness, key medical processes (such as gut surgery, caesarean sections, joint replacements, and chemotherapy for cancer) could become too dangerous to perform.

This incredible FAB technology is now available to us all. By adopting Frequency and Bioenergy approaches as your preferred medical healthcare treatment, you will be instrumental in implementing this new paradigm shift. So, buy or borrow devices, talk to friends who own them, use clinics that have invested in FAB healing modalities and seek out natural medicine. And if we choose not to—will it matter? Well yes, actually, this time it really will matter!

Our choice and voice will begin as a hum, building together as groups into a murmur and finally as millions choose FAB medicine it will result in a great song. It's time for humanity to wake up, thrive and ensure our collective survival. Employing what seems to be a radical shift of consciousness need be no more than reclaiming our humanity and using all the knowledge we have. Everyone will benefit, including the planet and all its lifeforms. I love win-win solutions, don't you?

Thank you for taking this journey with me, and I'm look forward hugely to meeting you online, at an event or through my other books!

With love and light
Paulette

Author's Note

This book is complete.

But my work is just beginning.

I want to reach out to all of you with ready hearts and minds who want to make the leap of consciousness and lift yourself to unknown heights of awareness; yet, remembering who you are and appreciating the simple things in life.

This morning my short walk around the hillside in Scotland brought many delicious gifts. I found an old plum tree on a foot path and filled my pockets with juicy, organic ripe fruits. We have picked some 15lb of blackberries (brambles) from the hedgerows and my mother is making five gallons of wine! Another picking and we made bramble jelly, all packed with goodness for the winter months. Mum is still using a recipe book she was given by her sister over fifty years ago, combining the wisdom of the WI (Women's Institute) ladies. It is splattered with five decades of fruit juices and is a most treasured possession.

Within a mile of the house, there are wild red currants which gave such a crop that we have made jelly to see us through a whole year. Last summer's discovery was an ancient gooseberry bush up against a wall, hidden amongst some nettles which gave 8lbs of sweet pink fruits, and a lot of scratches picking them. We had gooseberry crumble on Christmas day—enough to feed the whole family. Speaking of scratched arms and fingers, the next round of hedgerow miracle picking will be the sloes. Bitter, but when pricked, covered in gin and a bit of sugar makes the most incredible sloe gin! Forget the stuff in shops that tastes like almond essence. Go for the real thing and make your own.

Around the hamlet, tiny wild strawberries grow in abundance; they are utterly delicious. Raspberries are also found in the hedgerows but on mass in the local farms and we have three gallons of wine fermenting away beside the AGA (kitchen range). Oh, and seventeen pots of raspberry (raw) jam in the freezer. And in between all this, we found time to make yummy autumn chutney with apples plucked from our neighbour's trees.

Walking along some other country roads brought a new find: an incredible bush dripping with black currants. The elderberries are just ripening and my goodness the fungi/mushrooms are just everywhere in the fields and forests and pathways, even the golf courses! What a magical world. We don't have to go far to appreciate the abundance and beauty all around us. What do you have hidden in full sight near you?

I don't know if all these wild bushes and trees seeded themselves or if someone planted them years ago to help feed the poor folks working on the land, but what if you and I start to plant them? If every reader added to their parks, gardens and quiet roadsides these life-giving and nourishing plants, trees and bushes, the next generation will have so much waiting for them to pick as they wander past.

The tawny owls hooting kept me awake late into the night, and, as I listened, I wondered what they would say to all of us? Maybe they are asking us to wake up and enjoy the peace and softness right here under our noses. In nature, we find the hidden ways and are able to walk through the veil into all the realms of light.

You have the information within these pages to feed the goodness in your soul. Starting down this path of light will test you and many little pockets of old pain and fear may surface as they become illuminated by the rays of knowledge. The old saying, 'the truth will set you free' is relevant here or we can say 'the light will set you free' or 'authentic knowledge and its application will set you free'. Yes, it will, and you will know you are on the right track because of these simple guidelines:

1. When you do something—does it feel right in your heart?

2. Does it bring people, families, communities together (separation and isolation are methods that less evolved people use to control or manipulate others.)

3. Are you laughing, having fun and playing more? Can you feel innocence coming back?

4. Do things get easier, small miracles seem to happen and co-incidences follow you?

5. Are you spending more time in nature and being fuelled by its hidden power?

6. Do you have more energy, look healthier and feel strong deep inside?

7. Are you meeting lots of new people who also have big hearts and a different outlook?

Choosing to live with light and energy is one of the fastest ways to reach our full potential, heal all parts of ourselves and become a light to others.

We live in the most extraordinary time on Earth, where we have the potential to step into higher realms and bring heaven upon the earth. You are uniquely positioned to light a candle of hope and transformation. Only you can make that decision and become the one who helps, guides and leads others to the light.

Will you carry a torch for a new era where kindness, love and respect are the norm?

Separation does not exist in the realms of light and universal energy; we are all one and part of each other. We can use our individual power and gifts to add to the whole. Darkness cannot exist where there is light. There is an old tale from the Native Peoples of America where two wolves are fighting. A black one and a white one. The young warrior asks his grandmother, 'who will win?' And she replies, 'the one you feed'.

We are the caretakers of the earth—you and me. That's it. No one is coming to save us all and why try and go to another planet? We are living on the best planet there is.

Thank You

A big thank you to all my readers. This book wouldn't exist without it and it is by your word-of-mouth that the idea of FAB Health will spread.

For further, updated information, including more information on the next book, please visit my website.

www.pauletteagnew.com

Further Reading and Additional Materials

Look out for other books in the FAB series.

In the second book of this series, I show you how successful Frequency and Bioenergy clinics in Europe work to combine technology, cutting edge devices and natural healing methodologies. For those interested in finding alternatives to antibiotics and new models of health care, you will find this sequel invaluable. You will learn the protocols and combinations of devices and techniques used to treat daily health problems, along with Lyme, its co-infections and other chronic diseases.

For more information, visit www.pauletteagnew.com.

Beyond Fatigue—Online Programme

Paulette is uniquely positioned to help people suffering from Chronic Fatigue, Lyme disease and other conditions that leave you bed-ridden and incapacitated with pain, inflammation or exhaustion.

She has specialized in teaching therapeutic movement work, yoga, meditation and breathing for nearly thirty years. When Paulette contracted Borrelia and multiple coinfections, this led to her gradual decline in health with multiple systems affected, leading to a few years of being almost bedridden and confined to the house.

Initially she did not know what was causing the pain, insomnia, fatigue and numbness, but she refused to give up and tackled her illnesses with the tools she had. She knew that living a sedentary life would exacerbate her condition, not just physically, but also emotionally and mentally. Being trapped inside her body, watching it deteriorate and crash after a short walk around the garden, she decided to adapt and develop the techniques she knew. She adapted the self-help methods she taught in war zones and in corporate board rooms to suit her now bedridden state.

This unique action plan slowed the physical and mental degeneration during the illness and sped up recovery and the rebuilding of tissues as the Borrelia and co-infections were killed off. Paulette says, 'it's important to do something even when you feel you are powerless, exhausted and isolated from normal social and family interactions'.

When she got well, she decided to record all her best exercise routines and created this online programme. The ten classes are first of its kind. They are designed especially for people with limited mobility.

The programme is progressive, gentle and is designed to prevent crashing or burnout. The exercises begin lying down on the floor or in bed and gradually move to standing. Each class also has a short talk with tips, insights and methods to tackle the challenges and fears facing those with chronic fatigue, fibromyalgia and chronic diseases.

Recognised by doctors, Beyond Fatigue will help: increase energy flow, ignite positive feelings, maintain flexible joints and conserve muscle tone. You will learn simple but profound techniques to strengthen core stability, reduce back pain, etc. Details at www.beyondfatigue.com

"As a family doctor, I've always been sceptical about 'miraculous cures', but I have been so impressed by Paulette's recovery using this programme. It is clear to me that it can be of enormous benefit to people with chronic conditions and debilitating diseases such as fibromyalgia, chronic fatigue, Lyme, arthritis and any condition that stops people moving.

I can thoroughly recommend Beyond Fatigue to everyone who suffers from fatigue and exhaustion, whatever the cause."

–Dr Jane Fitzgerald MRCGP, UK.

www.beyondfatigue.com

Also by Paulette Agnew

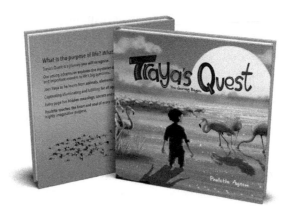

A spiritual odyssey written for children, but aimed for the enjoyment of all. Trayas's Quest touches upon life's most important lessons using captivating characters, luminous art and wilderness as surroundings.

Traya himself is a young Indian lad who has the gift of being able to hear and communicate with things and creatures many of us think don't have anything to say. Butterflies, pythons, spiders, the ocean, sun and moon all can beautifully communicate with each other and Traya can converse with them all!

He discovers that these friends of nature and the world have important lessons to teach him—all about Dharma—their reasons for being. As he meets his new friends, he starts to listen to his own heart and reflects upon his own Dharma. He finally decides that his purpose may just be what interconnects all beings: unconditional love.

This beautifully written story gives us a pause, causes us to consider our own Dharma and, most fundamentally, gives us a glimpse of the wonderful world we live in and how we all contribute to its wonderment. If you want to know why we are called human 'beings' and not human 'doings', explore Traya's world.

Is *Traya's Quest* a children's book, or is it a magical lesson for every single person who can read or tell its story? Whatever it is best called, it should be required reading for the entire world. Do yourself a favor and discover *Traya's Quest*. www.trayasquest.com

About the Author

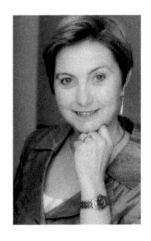

Paulette loves wilderness and nature and has worked in many parts of the world. Unknowingly, she contracted Lyme disease in Southern Sudan, which despite a ten-year battle to stay well, resulted in paralysis, cardiac problems, memory loss, extreme chronic fatigue and a close brush with death. Among her discoveries along the way was that the UK and US are behind Europe in treating Lyme, that sufferers can often feel alone or abandoned and those practitioners who (without endless drugs) can understand, diagnose and treat Lyme are rare. (She herself left her native UK to relocate to mainland Europe for treatment.)

Critically ill, Paulette decided to confront her condition head on with an initial four-month visit to a specialist Frequency and Bioenergtic (FAB) Medicine clinic. Through this experience, Paulette began to study and really understand how the body works at quantum, particle and light levels—how it becomes sick and how it can be healed. She reveals all with FAB Health in simple, concise language.

The unique approach offered at the European FAB clinic has created a paradigm shift in how we can look at healing on a global scale. It works, it's replicable, it's financially viable and it's enlightening. In her second book, she explains Frequency devices and their practical application for both personal and clinical use.

Paulette trained in Biochemistry, ran an outdoor pursuits school and is a prized motivational speaker. She is a spiritual mentor with a deep, lifelong belief in spiritual and holistic wellness. She has practiced and taught yoga and meditation for over twenty five years, openly sharing her love and mastery of the internal arts, altogether creating an unusual yet excellent background with which to tackle the subject. Her writing is clear, concise, forthright and humorous. After reading this book, readers will likely be able to envision a worldwide network of FAB clinics devoted to the treatment of Superbugs, Lyme and day to day health problems.

That possibility shines like a beacon of hope and Ms. Agnew's book is uniquely positioned to further that cause. For more information on FAB devices, interviews, coaching, online courses and more, visit **www.pauletteagnew.com**.

Acknowledgements

My eternal gratitude goes to Rogier for saving my life from horrendous and chronic Lyme Disease. His extraordinary insights, persistence and dedication to helping thousands of people goes beyond the call of duty. Liselotte Hennekam, thank you for being my rock and the best friend on this journey of healing and inner transformation.

Behind the scenes there are angels volunteering their skills to help get this message out to the world. Proof readers extraordinaire are Nigel Morrison and Ryan Currans. Beata Kozak came in at the final hour to project manage and kindly pushed me on to finalise the book, you are the best project manager in the world. This book would not have made it without you.

Other wonderful proof readers, technical advisors and editors include: Aubrey Kosa, David Kozak, Virginia Maxwell, Rory Weller, Rachel Baker-Searle, Barbara Lauger, David Franklin, Ewan McCabe, Christine Poland, Tamara Bell, Marcus Schmieke, Jerry Van den Bosch, Dorian Cook, Alan E. Baklayan, and Dr Elizabeth Davies. Chris Barrington my dearest friend and adopted big brother, thank you for a lifetime of love and quantum wisdom (and yes editing the physics!).

Anita Goswami, Savitri MacCuish, Gijs Bolomy, Marlene Mombers, Ineke de Hulster and many others, thank you for hosting me and driving me to the clinic over those initial four tough months. Sylvia Barrington, thank you for holding together my Yoga and Meditation School in Ireland when I was unable to walk or work. It takes good friends to help you through the dark times when there appears to be no light at the end of the tunnel.

I am grateful to my dear friend in Dubai, Jamal Almana, who has understood and supported this project from day one. You introduced me to some very special inventors and doctors in United Arab Emirates (UAE) who in turn opened my eyes to some really great science.

Thank you all for believing in this book.

Chris Ion, you are a very talented artist. Your humorous sketches are delightful.

In gratitude to Morgan James Publishing for seeing *FAB Health's* potential and bringing it to the wider public.

Much of the wisdom in this book comes from multiple contributors, scientists, healers, practitioners and explorers of frontier medicine, thank you all for your work and for being open to new ways of helping humanity heal and evolve.

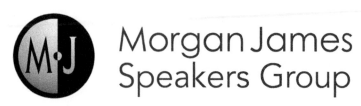

Morgan James
Speakers Group

↗ www.TheMorganJamesSpeakersGroup.com

We connect Morgan James published
authors with live and online events
and audiences who will benefit
from their expertise.

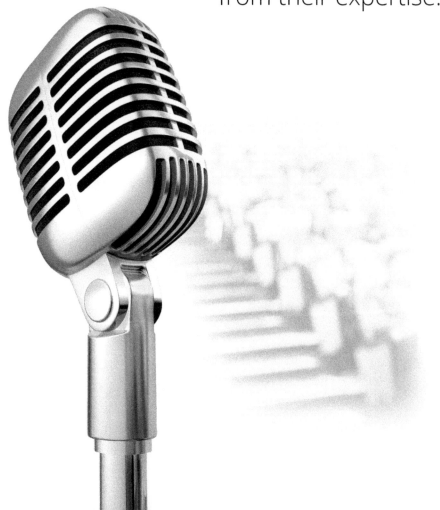

References

"Antimicrobial resistance." World Health Organization. Accessed October 27, 2017. http://www.who.int/mediacentre/factsheets/fs194/en/.

O'Neill, Jim. "Tackling Drug-Resistant Infections Globally: Final Report and Recommendations." Review on Antimicrobial Resistance. May 2016. Accessed October 27, 2017. https://amr-review.org/sites/default/files/160525_Final%20paper_with%20cover.pdf.

Introduction

Welcome to GOV.UK. Accessed October 27, 2017. https://www.gov.uk/government.

"WHO's first global report on antibiotic resistance reveals serious, worldwide threat to public health." WHO. Accessed October 27, 2017. http://www.who.int/mediacentre/news/releases/2014/amr-report/en/.

Chapter 2

Adam, Waldemar, and Giuseppe Cilento. Chemical and biological generation of excited states. New York: Academic Press, 1982.

Bajpai, R. P. "Quantum coherence of biophotons and living systems." NOPR: Home. May 01, 2003. Accessed October 27, 2017. http://nopr.niscair.res.in/handle/123456789/17068.

Bischof, Marco. Biophotonen: das Licht in unseren Zellen. Frankfurt am Main: Zweitausendeins, 2005.

Dürr, Hans-Peter, Fritz-Albert Popp, and Wolfram Schommers. What is life?: scientific approaches and philosophical positions. Singapore: World scientific, 2002.

Jinzhu), Chang Jiin-Ju (Zhang. "Physical properties of biophotons and their biological functions." NOPR: Home. May 01, 2008. Accessed October 27, 2017. http://nopr.niscair.res.in/handle/123456789/4474.

Klotter, Jule. "Light Cancer and Fritz-Albert Popp." Townsend Letter. Aug. & sept. 2010. Accessed October 27, 2017.

Popp, F.A, K.H Li, and Q. Gu. Recent advances in biophoton research and its applications. Singapore: World Scientific, 1992.

Rhesusplus. Biophotons - The Light in Our Cells. Accessed October 27, 2017. http://www.transpersonal.de/mbischof/englisch/webbookeng.htm.

Society, E. Research. "About the Coherence of Biophotons Fritz-Albert Popp International Institute of Biophysics (Biophotonics) Raketenstation, 41472 Neuss, Germany." Academia.edu. 1999. Accessed May 2017. http://www. academia.edu/1901658/About_the_Coherence_of_Biophotons_Fritz-Albert_Popp_International_Institute_of_Biophysics_Biophotonics_Raketenstation_41472_Neuss_Germany.

Takeda, M., M. Kobayashi, M. Takayama, S. Suzuki, T. Ishida, K. Ohnuki, T. Moriya, and N. Ohuchi. "Biophoton detection as a novel technique for cancer imaging." Cancer science. August 2004. Accessed October 27, 2017. https://www.ncbi.nlm.nih.gov/pubmed/15298728.

Popp, Fritz-Albert. 'About the Coherence of Biophotons,' Fritz-Albert Popp International Institute of Biophysics (Biophotonics) Raketenstation, 41472 Neuss, Germany. Published in "Macroscopic Quantum Coherence," Proceedings of an International Conference on the Boston University, Edited by Boston University and MIT, 1999.

Chapter 3

Electrons, photons, and the photo-electric effect. Accessed October 27, 2017. http://physics.bu.edu/~duffy/PY106/PhotoelectricEffect.html.

Pert, Candace B. Molecules of emotion: why you feel the way you feel. New York: Scribner, 2003.

Tennant, Jerry. Healing is voltage: the handbook. Irving, TX: Jerry Tennant, 2010.

Chapter 4

Lipton, Bruce H. The biology of belief: unleashing the power of consciousness, matter & miracles. Carlsbad, CA: Hay House, Inc., 2014.

Chapter 5

Andrade, A. C., C. Fernandes, L. Verghese, and C. Andrade. "Effect of negative ion atmospheric loading on cognitive performance in human volunteers." Indian journal of psychiatry. July 1992. Accessed October 27, 2017. https://www.ncbi.nlm.nih.gov/pubmed/21776128.

Chapter 6

http://www.item-bioenergy.com/infocenter/consciousintentionondna.pdf

Krueger, A. P., E. J. Reed, K. B. Brook, and M. B. Day. "Air ion action on bacteria." International Journal of Biometeorology 19, no. 1 (1975): 65-71. doi:10.1007/bf01459843.

Strachan, D., and J. Karnstedt. Negative Ions - Vitamins of the Air. Accessed May 2017. http://www.negativeionsinformation.org/ions_vitamins.html.

'Negative Ion Therapy for Depression.' Columbia University Technology Ventures, Technology #382, American Journal of Psychiatry. 2006; 163(12):2126-33.—Psychological Medicine. 2005; 35(7):945-55.—Journal of Alternative and Complementary Medicine. 1995; 1(1):87-92. http://innovation.columbia.edu/technologies/382_negative-ion-therapy-for-depression Accessed May 2017. http://www.cumc.columbia.edu/psjournal/archive/archives/jour_v19no1/light.html

'Your Body is Electrical and Runs on Electrons—NOT Sugar, Protein or Fat!' ACI Scholarly Blog Index, http://scholar.aci.info/view/14c4e82e3ab000e0009/14f4656d9f0000169 Accessed May 2017. https://www.newscientist.com/article/mg22329781-600-spark-of-life-revisited-thanks-to-electric-bacteria/

https://www.newscientist.com/article/dn25894-meet-the-electric-life-forms-that-live-on-pure-energy/

Chapter 7

Batmanghelidj, F. Your bodys many cries for water. Vienna, Virginia USA: Global Health Solutions, Inc., 2001.

Chen, Chi-Shuo, Wei-Ju Chung, Ian C. Hsu, Chien-Ming Wu, and Wei-Chun Chin. "Force field measurements within the exclusion zone of water." Journal of Biological Physics 38, no. 1 (2011): 113-20. doi:10.1007/s10867-011-9237-5.

Ho, Mae-Wan. Living rainbow H2O. Singapore: World Scientific Publ., 2012.

Hunt, Tam. "The rainbow and the worm: Establishing a new physics of life." Communicative & Integrative Biology. March 01, 2013. Accessed October 27, 2017. http://www.ncbi.nlm.nih.gov/pmc/articles/PMC3609844/.

Pollack, Gerald H. The fourth phase of water: beyond solid, liquid, and vapor. Seattle: Ebner and Sons, 2013.

Rohani, Mina, and Gerald H. Pollack. "Flow through Horizontal Tubes Submerged in Water in the Absence of a Pressure Gradient: Mechanistic Considerations." Langmuir 29, no. 22 (2013): 6556-561. doi:10.1021/la4001945.

Montagnier, et al. 'DNA Waves and Water,' Journal of Physics: Conference Series, Volume 306, Number 1, http://iopscience.iop.org/article/10.1088/1742-6596/306/1/012007/meta Accessed May 2017. http://iopscience.iop.org/article/10.1088/1742-6596/306/1/012007/meta

Davenas, E., Beauvais, F., Amara, J., et al. 'Human Basophil Degranulation Triggered by Very Dilute Antiserum Against IgE,' Nature 333, 816-818, 30 June 1988. https://www.ncbi.nlm.nih.gov/pubmed/2455231

Chapter 8

"Advanced research on the health benefit of reduced water." Trends in Food Science & Technology. November 09, 2011. Accessed October 27, 2017. http://www.sciencedirect.com/science/article/pii/S0924224411002408.

Chapter 9

Cousens, Gabriel. Conscious eating. Berkeley (Calif.): North Atantic Books, 2000.

Chapter 10

6, 2011 March. "Glutathione and the Methylation Cycle by Rich Van Konynenburg Ph.D." Phoenix Rising. April 21, 2012. Accessed May 2017. http://phoenixrising.me/treating-cfs-chronic-fatigue-syndrome-me/treating-chronic-fatigue-syndrome-mecfs-glutathione-and-the-methylation-cycle/simplified-treatment-approach-based-on-the-glutathione-depletion-methylation-cycle-block-pathogenesis-hypothesis-for-chronic-fatigue-syndrome-cfs-by-rich-van-konynenburg-ph-d.

Chapter 12

Ali, Yadollahpour, Rashidi Samaneh, and Fatemeh Kavakebian. "Applications of Magnetic Water Technology in Farming and Agriculture Development: A Review of Recent Advances." Current World Environment. Accessed May 2017. http://www.cwejournal.org/vol9no3/applications-of-magnetic-water-technology-in-farming-and-agriculture-development-a-review-of-recent-advances/.

Test. "Effects of Magnetic Water in Concrete • Aggregate Research International." Aggregate Research International. March 14, 2016. Accessed May 2017. https://www.aggregateresearch.com/news/effects-of-magnetic-water-in-concrete/.

Tkachenko, Yuri P. Mysteries of magnetic energies. Sharjah, UAE: Emirates Print. & Pub., 1995.

Chapter 13

"The Gut: Where Bacteria and Immune System Meet." Johns Hopkins Medicine, based in Baltimore, Maryland. Accessed May 2017. http://www.hopkinsmedicine.org/research/advancements-in-research/fundamentals/in-depth/the-gut-where-bacteria-and-immune-system-meet.

"Human Microbiome Project - Home." National Institutes of Health. Accessed May 2017. https://commonfund.nih.gov/hmp.

Chapter 17

McCabe, Ed. Flood Your Body With Oxygen. Energy Pubns Llc, 2009.

Roehm, D.C. 'The Bio Electron, Re-Examining the Work of Johanna Budwig,' Townsend Letter for Doctors and Patients, July1990, p.480.

Chapter 19

6, 2011 March. "Glutathione and the Methylation Cycle by Rich Van Konynenburg Ph.D." Phoenix Rising. April 21, 2012. Accessed May 2017. http://phoenixrising.me/treating-cfs-chronic-fatigue-syndrome-me/treating-chronic-fatigue-syndrome-mecfs-glutathione-and-the-methylation-cycle/simplified-treatment-approach-based-on-the-glutathione-depletion-methylation-cycle-block-pathogenesis-hypothesis-for-chronic-fatigue-syndrome-cfs-by-rich-van-konynenburg-ph-d.

Andrade, A. C., C. Fernandes, L. Verghese, and C. Andrade. "Effect of negative ion atmospheric loading on cognitive performance in human volunteers." Indian journal of psychiatry. July 1992. Accessed May 2017. https://www.ncbi.nlm.nih.gov/pubmed/21776128.

Carper, Jean. Stop aging now!: the ultimate plan for staying young and reversing the aging process. New York: HarperCollins, 1996.

"Curing Electromagnetic Hypersensitivity – My Review." ElectricSense. November 03, 2014. Accessed May 2017. http://www.electricsense. com/8862/curing-electromagnetic-hypersensitivity-my-review/.

Gutman, Jimmy, and Stephen Schettini. Glutathione (GSH): your bodys most powerful protector. Montréal: Kudo.ca Communications, 2002.

Lavelle, Marianne. "Mothers May Pass Lyme Disease to Children in the Womb." Scientific American. September 22, 2014. Accessed May 2017. https://www. scientificamerican.com/article/mothers-may-pass-lyme-disease-to-children-in-the-womb/.

"Press Release CDC Provides Estimate of Americans Diagnosed with Lyme Disease Each Year." Centers for Disease Control and Prevention. August 19, 2013. Accessed May 2017. https://www.cdc.gov/media/releases/2013/p0819-lyme-disease.html.

Publishing, Harvard Health. "Vitamin D and your health: Breaking old rules, raising new hopes." Harvard Health Publications. February 2007. Accessed May 2017. http://www.health.harvard.edu/newsletter_article/vitamin-d-and-your-health-breaking-old-rules-raising-new-hopes.

Soyka, Fred, and Alan Edmonds. The ion effect: how air electricity rules your life and health. Place of publication not identified: Bantam, 1991.

"The Difference Between Depression and Lyme Depression." Public Health Alert | Investigating Lyme Disease and Chronic Illness. November 15, 2014. Accessed May 2017. http://www.publichealthalert.org/the-difference-between-depression-and-lyme-depression.html.

"The Lyme Disease Challenge." ILADS. Accessed May 2017. http://www. ilads.org/ilads_news/2016/the-lyme-disease-challenge-%E2%80%9Cbites-back%E2%80%9D-and-raises-over-100000-to-support-lyme-disease/.

Sandor, S., Tache, Y., Somogyi, A. 'The Legacy of Hans Selye and the Origins of Stress Research: A Retrospective 75 Years After His Landmark Brief "Letter to the Editor" of Nature.' Stress, September 2012, 15(5), 472-478. DOI: 10.3109/10253890.2012.71091. http://selyeinstitute.org/wp-content/uploads/2013/06/TheLegacuyofHansSelyearticle.pdf

Interlandi, J. '"Messing With" the Blood-Brain Barrier May Be Key to Treating a Host of Diseases," Scientific American, June 2013. https://www. scientificamerican.com/article/messing-with-blood-brain-barrier-key-treating-host-diseases/

Effect of yoga on oxidative stress in elderly with grade-I hypertension: a randomized controlled study. Patil SG, Dhanakshirur GB et al. J Clin Diagn Res. 2014 Jul;8(7):BC04-7. https://www.ncbi.nlm.nih.gov/pubmed/25177555

http://apps.who.int/iris/bitstream/10665/163473/1/WHO_HSE_PED_AIP_2015.1_eng.pdf?ua=1&ua=1

http://who.int/bulletin/volumes/95/8/16-179648/en/